Challenges in
Medical Care

Challenges in Medical Care

Edited by Andrew Grubb

*School of Law and
Centre of Medical Law and Ethics
King's College, London, UK*

JOHN WILEY & SONS

Chichester · New York · Brisbane · Toronto · Singapore

Other Wiley editorial offices

John Wiley & Sons, Inc., 605 Third Avenue,
New York, NY 11158-0013, USA

Jacaranda Wiley Ltd, G.P.O. Box 859, Brisbane,
Queensland 4001, Australia

John Wiley & Sons (Canada) Ltd, 22 Worcester Road,
Rexdale, Ontario M9W 1L1, Canada

John Wiley & Sons (SEA) Pte Ltd, 37 Jalan Pemimpin 05-14,
Block B, Union Industrial Building, Singapore 2057

Library of Congress Cataloguing-in-Publication Data

Challenges in medical care / edited by Andrew Grubb.
    p.   cm.
    Includes bibliographical references and index.
    ISBN 0 471 93102 0
    1. Medical ethics. I. Grubb, Andrew.
    [DNLM: 1. Ethics, medical. 2. Legislation, Medical. W 50 C437]
    R724.C43 1992
    174'.2—dc20
    DNLM/DLC
    for Library of Congress   91-27615
                                                                        CIP

British Library Cataloguing in Publication Data

A catalogue record for this book is
available from the British Library

ISBN 0 471 93102 0

Typeset by Harper Phototypesetters Ltd, Northampton, England
Printed in Great Britain by Biddles Ltd, Guildford

Contents

Contributors

Trevor Clay CBE is first Vice President, International Council of Nurses and formerly General Secretary of the Royal College of Nursing.

Andrew Grubb is a Barrister, Senior Lecturer in Law and a Director of the Centre of Medical Law and Ethics, King's College London.

Most Rev and Rt Hon John Habgood is Archbishop of York.

Ian Kennedy is Professor of Medical Law and Ethics, Head and Dean of the School of Law and Executive Director of the Centre of Medical Law and Ethics, King's College London.

Gayle Rawlings is a Consultant in Radiation Oncology, Princess Margaret Hospital, Toronto, Canada.

David Seedhouse is Head of the Unit for the Study of Health Care Ethics, University of Liverpool.

Margaret Stacey is Emeritus Professor of Sociology, University of Warwick.

Ellen Stein is a Research Fellow at the Nuffield Department of Obstetrics and Gynaecology, John Radcliffe Hospital, Oxford.

Jenifer Wilson-Barnett is Professor of Nursing Studies and a Director of the Centre of Medical Law and Ethics, King's College London.

Preface

This is the sixth volume of essays on medical law and ethics published by the Centre of Medical Law and Ethics at King's College, London. The volume consists of two groups of papers. First, there are those which saw the light of day as part of the Centre's Lent Lecture series in 1990 (Habgood, Grubb and Clay). Secondly, the remaining papers were commissioned to represent a cross-section of some of the important issues in the area during 1990–1991 (Kennedy and Grubb, Rawlings, Stein, Stacey, Seedhouse and Wilson-Barnett). Some of the papers return to problems and controversies that have long challenged medical law and medical ethics. Others show how new issues are constantly arising out of developments in medical care.

The diversity of subject matter reflects the breadth of issues which the health care professionals must face in their day to day working lives. The papers take a reflective view on these issues and prompt the reader to question these developments and some of the challenges which will be faced in the 1990s.

Perhaps the golden thread that can be detected is the need to question process and substance as they evolve. The need for responsibility, accountability and respect for (individual) human rights can be seen in each of the contributions, however the particular debate is concluded.

It is hoped that this volume, as with previous ones, raises these questions and allows those whose agenda involves the formulation of public policy—which, of course, is all of us—to keep fully informed.

Andrew Grubb
King's College
London

HIV and AIDS: discrimination and the challenge for human rights*

Ian Kennedy and Andrew Grubb

Introduction

The sick are commonly the object of adverse discrimination in many countries. Their status as sick may mean that they are unable to work, or organise their lives, or are dependent on others. As a consequence, they often find themselves living in circumstances of relative poverty without proper health care or support from social services. They also often find themselves powerless to effect any improvement in their position, either because they are sick or because their illness prevents them from organising and lobbying effectively. The mentally ill are a striking example of such a group. If societies purport to embrace the approach to the care of the mentally ill which contemplates care in "the community" rather than in a secure institution (an *asylum* in its original and important meaning), and then fail actually to provide the resources for such care, adverse discrimination inevitably follows.

The stigmatising of the sick and adverse discrimination against them is more marked in some circumstances than others. To a large extent, this reflects the prevailing societal view of the particular illness and the sufferer. Susan Sontag in her book *Illness as Metaphor*[1] contrasts the romanticism which surrounded

---

* This article is based on a paper delivered by Professor Kennedy to the 7th Colloquium on Human Rights organised by the Council of Europe, Copenhagen, May 1990.

affliction with tuberculosis in the 19th century, with the revulsion many feel about cancer, and hence, she argues, cancer sufferers in the 20th century. The sufferer can be stigmatised on a number of grounds. It may be because of what the illness does to the sufferer whether physically or mentally. It may be because of the risk of acquiring a particular disease. It may be because of the alleged immorality of conduct by which the illness was contracted. Syphilis exemplifies all these forms of stigmatisation, as do other venereal diseases, albeit to a lesser extent. Leprosy is another example which has been with us for many hundreds of years, indeed in Biblical times. Common to both of these conditions, and others, is a pattern of discrimination involving segregation, shunning, isolation and attendant marginalisation and consequent poverty and desperation.

HIV infection and AIDS are another example of this sad history of ignorance, incomprehension, prejudice and discrimination. They pose the same problems for societies.[2] The question for us is whether, now that there exist a battery of provisions for the protection of human rights at both national and international level, sufferers will fare better than their predecessors. Alternatively, will prejudice and fear swamp commitment to human rights and produce another chapter in the history of man's intolerance of his fellow man?

The UK response to the AIDS crisis

To examine the extent to which the UK has learned from history, we intend to do the following: first, to identify areas of possible discrimination against those with AIDS or who are HIV positive and secondly, to describe the current state of the law and practice in these areas.

What has been the response of the UK to AIDS and HIV infection? From the point of view of human rights, it can be said that the record of the UK has been very good indeed until relatively recently. There is recent evidence of a certain loss of nerve among those directing the Government's efforts. This arises, it is submitted, from a hardening of opinion among what is called the 'moral majority' and the acceptance of this view at the centre of Government.

The justification for commending the UK's response lies in the courageous early decision that AIDS and HIV infection were best dealt with as a public health issue.[3] Equally important, health education, health promotion and persuasion were to be the focuses of the Government's response.[4] The emphasis above all was on voluntariness and trust. Nothing of a compulsory nature was to be done, not only out of an abstract respect for rights but also for good pragmatic reasons: the epidemic could only be controlled if those who were already ill and those at risk could be persuaded to come forward for help. Anything which might frighten people away was therefore to be avoided. Thus, matters such as confidentiality, voluntary testing, explicit health education and counselling were stressed. It is difficult to know to what extent, if at all, the policies adopted by the UK Government have affected the incidence of AIDS and HIV positivity. There is a strong suspicion, however, that they have been instrumental in ensuring that the epidemic has been relatively well contained so far.

We referred earlier to a loss of nerve in recent Government responses to the epidemic. The evidence for this includes the refusal to underwrite the costs of an enquiry into sexual behaviour, so important in assessing and designing preventive and educative measures (the research has since been taken over by a non-governmental agency). Also, there has been a move away from more explicit health information and television campaigns towards more bland (and, some would say, less successful) broadcasts. Then, there has been the failure of Government to pass legislation preventing discrimination in the work place and its failure effectively to control possible discrimination by the insurance industry, which seriously affects perceptions about access to insurance and financial assistance for housing. Finally, and most significantly, has been the launching of a programme of testing blood without consent on an anonymised basis for epidemiological purposes.

Each of these more recent developments has significance from the point of view of human rights, whether it is the right to receive true and adequate information on which to base decisions about health and lifestyle, the right to housing and to work, or the right to health care.[5] Putting aside for the moment a detailed consideration of any one of these, they are all relevant here to suggest a wider point. The strength of a society's commitment to human rights often depends on nothing more than a set of perceptions held by the members of that society.

Preservation and protection of human rights depend on the belief that they are taken seriously. The merest suspicion that they are not will already alienate the weakest and most vulnerable, and thereby already begin to undermine their rights. It will also give encouragement to those elements in society who are always ready to feed on and encourage prejudice and consequent discrimination. Thus, the public posture, the public utterances of a society and its government are at one level critical in preventing or promoting discrimination.

It would be wrong not to note that the public utterances concerning AIDS and HIV infection emanating from bodies such as the Department of Health and the General Medical Council (the body which *inter alia* regulates the conduct of doctors) have, by and large, been steadfastly committed to the preservation of respect for the individual and his human rights. Two examples will suffice. The first concerns a doctor's duty to HIV positive patients or those who suffer from AIDS. In a significant step in May 1988, the GMC stated[6] that:

" . . . it is unethical for a registered medical practitioner to refuse treatment, or investigation for which there are appropriate facilities, on the ground that the patient suffered, or may suffer, from a condition which exposes the doctor to personal risk."

Conduct which is unethical could amount to serious professional misconduct and thereby attract disciplinary action against a doctor. In reaffirming an HIV patient's basic human right to treatment the GMC went further and stated[7] that:

"[it] is equally unethical for a doctor to withhold treatment from any patient on the basis of a moral judgement that the patient's activities or lifestyle might have contributed to the condition for which treatment was being sought."

Prejudice and judgmental considerations are not to take precedence over the patient's right to treatment. In any event, if proper precautions are taken to avoid risk-related contacts, the likelihood that a doctor's health would be jeopardised by treating an infected patient is minimal.[8]

In another statement issued in November 1989 the GMC again reaffirmed the rights of HIV infected individuals, in this case health care workers. Here, however, the interests of patients and doctors require a delicate balance to be achieved. The statement arose from the concern of some that HIV infected doctors might be jeopardising the health of their patients by continuing in practice. While it is conceivable that this could occur, there is currently no hard evidence of its ever occurring.[8a] With proper limitations on practice and if care is taken by the doctor or other health care worker to minimise risk-related contacts with patients, e.g. exposing them to blood, then the right of the doctor to continue his work does not prejudice the patient.[9] The GMC concluded that it would be unethical for a doctor to put his patients at risk if he knew or believed he was infected but that in consultation with a colleague he could often modify his behaviour and avoid such risks, perhaps by limiting the scope of his practice.

In both these instances we see the GMC striving to recognise and preserve the human rights of HIV infected individuals. This sensitive and informed approach is exemplary.

Discrimination

In general terms, we can divide discrimination into (1) that which is adverse to an individual, either himself or as a member of a group, and (2) that which shows preference to an individual himself or as a member of a group, thereby adversely affecting all others. The latter category of discrimination is usually overlooked in the context of AIDS and HIV, but there are a number of points which should be carefully considered. Obviously, however, it is the former category that attracts more attention.

1. Adverse discrimination

(a) Health care

(i) Access: Health care is a basic human right and one which will be of considerable importance to AIDS patients as their condition worsens. We have already seen the response of the GMC to reports that health care was being denied to HIV infected patients. Maintaining access to the best possible health care for AIDS patients is an important social goal.

(ii) HIV antibody testing and issues of consent:[10] Knowledge of HIV status may be important to the patient, to health care workers or society at large. Notwithstanding that the knowledge is of general significance, respect for the patient's right to self-determination, however, requires that his blood only be tested for HIV infection if he has voluntarily and explicitly consented to the test. In other words, a doctor must inform a patient of his intention to test his blood for HIV prior to taking the sample. The patient must have the right to refuse given the significant social, economic and emotional consequences which a determination of HIV positivity may have for an individual. In May 1988 the GMC approved a statement which recognised the patient's right to know that his blood was to be tested for HIV infection.[11] Only in exceptional circumstances where it is not possible to obtain prior consent and a test is imperative in order to secure the safety of another would a doctor be justified according to the GMC in testing without *explicit consent.*[12]

English law may well reflect this ethical view which accords respect to the HIV patient's right to know and choose whether to consent to the HIV test. Failure to obtain explicit consent to test could well give rise to actions in battery and negligence.[13]

One aspect of testing in particular has given rise to some controversy in the UK.[14] Anonymised testing of blood which has been taken from patients for other purposes is claimed by some to be a valid means of obtaining epidemiological data to assist the Government in the formulation of public health policy to record and contain the spread of infection. In January 1990 the Government introduced a scheme of anonymised testing despite the opposition of the Royal College of Nursing and the Social Services Committee of the House of Commons. The scheme involves the use of an *aliquot* of blood taken for other purposes, which is then anonymised and tested for HIV infection. The scheme is optional and a patient may choose not to participate. Contrary to practice in other areas, however, e.g. tissue donation, and contrary to the various statements requiring express consent for testing, the patient will be assumed to consent to participate in the scheme unless she acts otherwise. The Government provides leaflets and posters at surgeries, clinics and hospitals which call attention to the scheme and the opportunity to opt out.[15]

A number of ethical arguments, which reflect human rights concerns, can be raised against anonymised testing.[16] First, it abandons the principle of voluntariness and openness hitherto endorsed by Government as the only proper means of respecting individuals' rights.

Thus, it undermines the desired objective of sensible public health policy which is to avoid driving those infected with HIV "underground" out of fear of reprisals if found to be positive, thereby further endangering public health.

Secondly, it means that by anonymising a blood sample, a doctor thereby subjugates the interests of his patient to those of society without the patient's explicit agreement, since thereafter, whatever the patient's condition, the doctor cannot respond since he has abandoned the patient. Thirdly, it results in the doctor being prevented from learning about his patient's condition and thereby assisting him. In view of the developments in the use of AZT and other compounds as a treatment to delay the progress of disease, the doctor may be denied the opportunity to offer real help to his patient. Fourthly, it produces a conflict between two public health goals. While epidemiological knowledge is obtained, the health of the population is put at risk since failure to identify an individual as HIV positive may put a spouse or future sexual partner at risk and thereby further the spread of the epidemic. Finally, bad science is bad ethics. A scheme of anonymised testing may be an invalid scientific method for obtaining valuable epidemiological data for the following three reasons. The information about the patient is not specific enough. The information obtained will not allow real knowledge of the spread and scope of the epidemic and so not permit the very planning the scheme is designed to facilitate. Further, because the samples are anonymised it will not be known whether the individual was, for example, an intravenous drug user, a homosexual or promiscuous heterosexual. Finally, the information, relating as it does to a particular limited time-frame, offers a snapshot of the condition of the population. A true picture will only emerge if the exercise is repeatedly done with a similar population, e.g. pregnant women or college students. However, the knowledge of the prevalence within these groups may not necessarily assist in formulating policy on a society-wide basis.

Sound public policy would pull us in a different direction away from anonymised testing to voluntary testing across a broader range of individuals. There is no reason to believe that properly informed individuals would not cooperate in such a scheme provided the Government was prepared to remove the obstacles currently raised by insurance companies (see later). Concern for human rights and respect for persons would, as a consequence, be better served by voluntary prevalence testing of this sort, accompanied by explicit consent and appropriate counselling prior to testing.[17]

(b) Employment There are two areas of employment law which particularly raise concerns about human rights and discrimination—recruitment and dismissal.

(i) Recruitment: in general, English law does not provide a remedy to a person who is refused employment because of some discriminatory attitude by an employer. There are two exceptions to this—sex discrimination[18] and racial discrimination.[19]

An employer may, therefore, choose not to employ a person who refuses to submit to an HIV antibody test. On the face of it, English law provides no remedy for this form of discrimination. The unfairness of the practice and its infringement of an individual's human rights cannot be justified by reference to the risk of transmission to others and the unsuitability of such a person for the job he seeks. Even if someone is HIV positive, rarely will a job carry a risk of transmission, though there may be a hypothetical risk in the health care sector. Equally untenable is the proposition that whether asymptomatic or not he will, for reasons having only to do with his HIV status, necessarily be incapable of working. Ill-health in the future is, of course, a different matter and may, if the individual is absent from work for sufficiently long periods, justify dismissal.

It could be argued that discrimination against HIV positive persons amounts to *indirect* discrimination on the grounds of sex since it has the effect of singling out men because of the link between HIV infection and homosexual men. Some support for this can be seen in the action taken by the Equal Opportunities Commission (EOC) in January 1987 against the airline Dan-Air.[20] The company had a policy of not employing men as temporary cabin staff. The company sought to defend its policy by claiming that there was a prevalence of homosexuality amongst male cabin staff and that there was a consequent danger to passengers from HIV infection if an accident occurred at work. The argument is, of course, spurious. Even if there were any incidence of HIV positivity amongst male cabin staff, the risk of transmission to passengers would be so remote as not to warrant consideration. The EOC issued a non-discrimination notice under section 67 of the Sex Discrimination Act 1975 requiring the company to change its recruitment practices.

Notwithstanding this example, it can be argued that it may be "wishful thinking about what the law ought to do rather than what it actually does" to apply the indirect discrimination provisions of the 1975 Act.[21] First, the link between homosexual practices and HIV is established but it is only one mode of transmission. Discriminating against individuals with HIV may not single out men at all. Secondly, discrimination on grounds of homosexuality is not unlawful and any potential employer could readily resort to this reason for non-employment. Thirdly, indirect discrimination may be justified. The test is an objective one permitting that which is "reasonably necessary". Hence "[a] refusal to employ someone HIV-positive because of the opposition and disruption which the recruitment of such an individual would be likely to cause among existing staff and customers might be defended on objective grounds".[22]

(ii) Dismissal: once an individual is employed English law provides greater protection. Apart from the common law principles of contract, the statutory scheme is the Employment Protection (Consolidation) Act 1978. This gives employees (subject to certain threshold conditions, e.g. two years' employment) a right not to be unfairly dismissed. Unfair dismissal may occur when an employer lacks a *substantive* ground for the dismissal within the Act or, where he does, he proceeds in a *procedurally* unfair manner. If an employer breaches the contract between him and the employee, then the employee may be able to resign and claim that he was constructively dismissed.

Two issues arise: first, can an employee claim unfair dismissal because he refuses an HIV antibody test; and secondly, would it be lawful to dismiss an employee on the basis of his HIV status?

Refusal of HIV test: in the absence of an express term in the contract of employment, employers cannot require an employee to undergo an HIV antibody test. Two possible exceptions to this are where the employment carries great responsibility and fitness to work may be prejudiced by the individual's HIV status, e.g. airline pilots or, perhaps, health care workers. Even these seem somewhat questionable if the employee is asymptomatic (in the case of the pilot) or proper precautions to protect others are taken (in the case of the health care worker). The other exception relates to employers' medical plans which call for a medical examination. Here HIV testing may be carried out as a condition to joining the plan. However, it is arguable that the results of the test are confidential and not subject to disclosure to the employer (see section on "privacy" below).

Beyond these situations it is arguable that an employee could claim he was unfairly dismissed if an employer dismissed him, or took other deleterious action and the employee resigned, wholly on the ground of his refusal to consent to testing. Such an action by the employer would be a breach of the implied term of mutual trust and confidence between employee and employer which is part of an employment contract. No case exists in the UK concerning HIV but in relation to a case where a doctor was suspended for refusing to undergo a medical examination, the Court of Appeal in *Bliss* v. *South East Thames RHA*[23] said:

> "It would be difficult, in this particular area of employment law, to think of anything more calculated to destroy the relationship of confidence and trust which ought to exist between employer and employee than without reasonable cause to require a consultant surgeon to undergo a medical . . . and to suspend him from hospital on his refusing to do so."

Of course (as the court made plain), the reason for the employer's action is crucial. We shall shortly return to this in the context of pressure from other employees or customers to dismiss the individual.

Legality of dismissal: whether it would be lawful to dismiss an employee who is HIV positive will turn upon the particular circumstances. The dismissal (or other action which leads the employee to resign) must be reasonable to be fair. A number of points need to be made in relation to this. First, an employer has both common law and statutory duties to take reasonable care for his employees' safety, including the provision of a proper and safe work environment. This would justify the employer in taking precautions to minimise or eliminate any risk (if it exists) of transmission of HIV to other workers. Generally, of course, there will be no such risk, though this need not always be the case. HIV positive employees are under an obligation to comply with these reasonable requirements and a failure to do so may justify dismissal.

What, however, if the employer chooses to dismiss the employee because of pressure from other employees or customers? Employees who are HIV positive could be the subject of harassment and unfair prejudice. An employer could not, without more, dismiss an employee in these circumstances. Much will turn upon the particular situation but an employer would have to consider relocating the complaining employees or the HIV positive employee to other suitable work. Equally the employer would have to attempt to lay to rest unfounded suspicions of the risk of infection.[24] However, if all fails, *dismissal could be lawful.*[25] It has been said that "as a matter of public policy, such pressure should be disregarded when it takes the form of prejudice against AIDS".[26] Nevertheless, it is likely that UK employment law will recognise that tribunals and courts in determining the reasonableness of an employer's conduct may mirror the prejudices of society instead of attempting to set higher standards than currently exist.[27]

The current law of employment does not, therefore, adequately safeguard the rights of HIV positive employees. The issue of confidentiality is also important in this context but we defer comment until later. To strengthen UK legislation two proposals have been made to protect an individual's rights. First, in 1989 an amendment to the (then) Employment Bill would have outlawed discrimination against HIV positive individuals in recruitment, employment and dismissal. Secondly, in 1987 the Terrence Higgins Trust, the leading charitable organisation concerned with AIDS, drafted an amendment to the unfair dismissal legislation of 1978 which would have made it unfair to dismiss someone simply on the basis of HIV status.[28] Neither proposal became law.

(c) Insurance The particular concern here is with the provision of life assurance.[29] Other forms of insurance, e.g. health insurance, also raise issues that relate to HIV infected

individuals and AIDS sufferers. It is increasingly becoming the case that health insurance excludes cover for any condition related to HIV infection or AIDS.

However, it is the availability of life assurance and the process of screening applicants for such assurance which generates the greatest concern for human rights and discrimination. It is important to notice at the outset that in the UK the insurance industry is not specifically regulated by Government.

In the UK, the insurance industry has attempted to identify two groups of individuals: first, those who are HIV positive, and secondly, those who are at risk of being infected because they are in a high risk group. The former will be excluded from obtaining life assurance, the latter may be also or, at least, they may be charged higher premiums.

Life assurance coverage is particularly important because 70 per cent of mortgages in the UK are secured by means of an endowment mortgage. Availability of life assurance is, therefore, closely related to an individual's ability to own a home.

Insurance contracts impose upon those who seek coverage a duty to answer truthfully all questions asked and to disclose all "material facts".[30] An individual's duty is only to disclose what he or she knows. As Fletcher Moulton LJ stated in *Joel* v. *Law Union Assurance Co*[31]

"The duty is a duty to disclose, and you cannot disclose what you do not know. The obligation to disclose, therefore, necessarily depends on the knowledge you possess . . . Your opinion of the materiality of that knowledge is of no moment. If a reasonable man would have recognised that it was material to disclose the knowledge in question, it is no excuse that you did not recognise it to be so."

In view of the importance that insurance companies place upon an individual's HIV status and potential for exposure to HIV, relevant information known to the individuals would constitute "material facts" because a reasonably prudent insurance company would wish to know the information.[32] Failure to answer truthfully may well result in the insurance company not honouring the contract (quite lawfully) on the death of the individual.[33]

The procedure recommended by the Association of British Insurers since 1986 for obtaining assurance is as follows:

1. Application form containing questions designed to elicit information as to whether the individual has ever been advised about AIDS or has had an HIV antibody test.
2. A supplementary questionnaire explicitly seeking information on whether the individual has been tested, received medical advice in relation to AIDS and further, whether the individual falls within a risk group, defined as homosexual men, bisexual men, intravenous drug users, haemophiliacs or sexual partners of any of these.
3. In the light of the above, further pursuit of information from the individual's general practitioner including details of lifestyle. Additionally, the individual may be required to have an HIV antibody test.

If an individual is HIV positive or refuses an antibody test he will be declined insurance. This may occur if the individual's test proves negative but he is in a high risk group. Alternatively, in this latter situation, an insurance policy may be issued but at a significantly higher premium.

A number of human rights concerns surface. First, is it proper to seek (and use) information about prior negative HIV testing? The House of Commons Social Services Committee thought not.[34] It is an unwarranted invasion of privacy. Furthermore, to disadvantage individuals on the basis of their past history of having been tested may have the effect of discouraging others from voluntarily seeking advice, counselling and testing. Sound public health policy should *encourage* responsibility in potential sufferers both out of a concern for their own health and the health of others. The perceived effect which even a negative test may have on an individual's future insurability is likely, however, to prejudice the achievement of this public health goal.

Secondly, there is a danger in identifying particular groups as representing potentially higher risks for insurance purposes. Not only is eliciting information concerning sexual orientation problematic and raises concerns about privacy. (In the US such questions have been outlawed by many state legislatures.[35]) But also sexual orientation alone is not an indicator of higher risk and so is discriminatory without a sound basis. The Government's blood donor screening programme illustrates the need to identify with precision the group at risk so as to eliminate the possibility of unjustified discrimination. No longer are homosexual men *per se* a high risk group—sexual contact must be established. At a more fundamental level, it is conduct which creates risk rather than membership of a particular group. This is the issue from the perspective of human rights.

Thirdly, the insurers' condition requiring testing for HIV of those considered at risk is unlikely to be abandoned. Safeguards are, therefore, essential to protect individual rights, such as the need for consent, counselling on HIV and on the consequences of a negative or positive test result, disclosure of the report to the individual[36] and the maintenance of confidentiality in the report. Confidentiality is essential and it can only be ensured if strict practices are adopted within the insurance industry to restrict dissemination of HIV test results even within a company.

It remains a matter of debate whether these matters can satisfactorily be dealt with by the insurance industry. Even if they can, it may be that in a matter of such importance, legislative intervention is called for. This has been the case in some American jurisdictions.[37] Indeed, a case could be made for arguing that the state may have a duty to those otherwise denied access to insurance (and, therefore, in the case of life cover, a home) to provide an alternative source of funds from which to gain insurance cover.

(d) Privacy   Throughout the discussion so far, issues have been raised which go to the heart of concern for an individual and his rights. At the heart is the right of privacy, which includes, in this context, the freedom to choose treatment, to refuse testing and to determine what information concerning him should be known and who should have access to it.[38] Under the specific heading of privacy, we wish to concentrate particularly on this last point. It highlights immediately the need for confidentiality of information relating to an individual's HIV status.[39] It arises in relation to all the areas considered so far: medical treatment, employment and insurance coverage.

The importance accorded to the obligation of confidence is well-established.[40] Respect for persons and their right to privacy support a strong (though not absolute) obligation not to disclose information relating to an individual's HIV status and a consequent expectation in the individual.

The GMC in its statement of May 1988 recognises the importance of this obligation in health care. Similarly, the law of the UK recognises the public interest in the confidentiality of medical information.[41] In relation to sexually transmitted diseases (probably including HIV infection and AIDS) the health carer's duty in law is stated in the National Health Service (Venereal Diseases) Regulations 1974.[42] In relation to HIV, in *X* v. *Y*, Rose J. expressed the public interest justifying confidentiality as follows:[43]

"In the long run, preservation of confidentiality is the only way of securing public health; otherwise doctors will be discredited as a source of education, for future patients will not come forward if doctors are going to squeal on them. Consequently, confidentiality is vital to secure public as well as private health, for unless those infected come forward they cannot be counselled and self-treatment does not provide the best care; opportunistic infections such as shortness of breath and signs of disease in the nervous system . . . are better detected and responded to by observation, investigation, and management in hospital."

Although referring to health care, the interests that the judge recognises are no less significant elsewhere when information of an individual's HIV status is obtained. It is a sad fact that prejudice, the basis of much discrimination, is still associated with HIV and AIDS. A failure to preserve and protect patients' confidences could lead to their being seriously disadvantaged socially and economically in society. Further, as the judge indicates, such a failure may result in patients being reluctant to seek testing or medical help and could thereby prejudice their health, the health of others and, ultimately, society as a whole.

The obligation of confidence is not absolute but, to give due weight to these compelling arguments of public policy, any disclosure should be exceptional.[44] The GMC in its statement of May 1988 accepts this and identifies two possible exceptions—where the disclosure is to the patient's health carers and where it is to the patient's spouse or sexual partner. Both of these are, in effect, set out as exceptions to the duty of confidentiality in the 1974 Regulations.[45]

In the case of disclosure to another health carer, for example the patient's GP, the GMC accepts that knowledge is necessary for the treatment of the individual. However, it is by no means clear that disclosure is justifiable if the patient, once asked (and in our view he must be asked), refuses permission to pass on to his GP the results of an HIV antibody test. Arguably, once the patient has been counselled about the problems that might be faced by a GP treating him without knowledge, he is entitled to have his privacy respected.[46]

If it could be validly argued that the other health carer would be placed at risk if unaware of the patient's condition, disclosure might be justified. But, this would be on the basis of protecting the doctor and not out of a concern for the patient's health interests. Rarely, however, will such a serious risk exist providing the doctor already ensures that the recommended precautions are taken irrespective of known HIV status.[47]

Let us now turn to the other exception. Where disclosure is necessary to protect another from a *serious and identifiable risk of infection*, then the patient's confidence *may* be broken. The most common situation where this could arise would be where an HIV positive patient informs a doctor that he does not intend to adopt "safer sex" practices and the doctor believes that the patient's known sexual partner will as a consequence be exposed to a real risk of infection. The specificity of the risk and the person at risk may justify disclosure.[48] UK law would most likely reflect this position providing, as always, that the doctor had fully counselled the patient on the risks of transmission, how to avoid them and had sought his permission to inform the sexual partner.[49] In this exceptional case the patient's privacy rights would give way to the more pressing interests of the sexual partner and the public interest in preventing the spread of the infection. The doctor will certainly have a discretion to warn the sexual partner. It may even be that he will have a legal duty to do so.[50]

The discussion has centred upon health care but the tensions between the privacy rights of the individual and the interests of others can be seen in other contexts.[51] For example, an employer may claim the right to inform co-employees of the HIV status of an employee. Arguably this could only be justified if a serious risk of transmission existed (which is most unlikely).

(e) Freedom of movement Two aspects of freedom of movement call for specific mention—immigration policy and public health provisions.

(i) Immigration: In recent years there have been reports that HIV infected persons were refused entry to the US because of the

alleged risk which they posed to public health through the spread of the infection. The US currently denies entry visas to HIV infected individuals except for temporary visits to, for example, conferences.[52] Such a policy lacks any basis in terms of rational analysis and presents a serious challenge to an individual's human rights, representing, as it does, a policy born of prejudice. The policy of the UK Government, on the other hand, is that HIV infected persons or AIDS sufferers will not be refused entry on the grounds of public health. Medical grounds can justify a refusal of entry to a visitor, and an immigration officer may refer a visitor to a medical inspector. Nevertheless, this procedure is not used to deny entry to HIV infected individuals. Public health needs do not call for such discriminatory action. The World Health Organisation in a Report in March 1987 following a meeting of experts[53] concluded that a general screening programme of international travellers was unfeasible because of the enormity of the task and, perhaps, more importantly, because it served no public health goal. The danger posed by travellers was no greater than the danger posed by residents. The idea that any country could keep HIV outside its borders is, in the reality of the 1990s, fanciful. HIV is already all around us. Viruses need no passports and respect no boundaries. The Report concluded:[54]

"The routes of HIV transmission have been documented to be the same throughout the world. Therefore, the behaviours that put individuals at risk of acquiring HIV are similar worldwide. Preventative measures against HIV are also the same worldwide, regardless of whether the individual is a traveller or a resident of a given country . . . Educational material should be made available for international travellers to increase awareness of how HIV is transmitted and how it can be prevented."

(ii) Public health: Perceived public health needs led the UK Government in 1985 to apply some of the provisions of the Public Health (Control of Disease) Act 1984 to AIDS.[55] The 1984 Act is concerned with public health needs in relation to those notifiable diseases listed in the Act such as cholera, plague, relapsing fever, smallpox and typhus.[56] Its provisions make significant inroads into an individual's rights by vesting in the responsible Government bodies extensive powers to control and combat the spread of disease. However, the 1988 Regulations

only apply (with some modifications) five provisions in the 1984 Act to AIDS; sections 35 (medical examination), 37 (removal to hospital), 38 (detention in hospital), 43 (death in hospital), and 44 (isolation of the body). Importantly, the Regulations do not make AIDS or HIV infection a notifiable disease. Indeed, it is significant that the Regulations only apply to AIDS; the Act is *not* extended to cover HIV itself. It is not entirely clear why provisions justified on public health grounds do not extend to HIV infected persons. It could be said that the Regulations are thereby made at best incoherent.

Before turning to the detail of the provisions themselves, it is clear that the Act provides some protection for individual rights by only permitting action to be taken under the Act after a judicial determination and subsequent order. Before sections 35, 37 or 38 apply, an order must be obtained from a Justice of the Peace. However, the Justice of the Peace may if he deems it necessary make an order under the Act without hearing the individual who is to be the subject of the order. There is a right of appeal under the Act to the Crown Court.

Medical examination: Section 35 permits a medical examination (without an individual's consent) if:

1. there is reason to believe he is suffering from AIDS, and
2. it is expedient to examine him in his own interests or the interests of his family or the public generally, and
3. any doctor under whose care he is, consents.

The section authorises a medical *examination* but not *treatment*. A medical examination would, of course, ordinarily include a test to detect the presence of the disease. It would be most significant if a doctor (albeit after a court appeal) could carry out an HIV antibody test without an individual's consent. But, the section *as it applies to HIV* does not allow a doctor to do this. Section 35 as is set out in the 1984 Act does permit non-consensual testing because it applies not only to a patient who is believed to have the notifiable disease but also to the patient who is believed to be ''carrying an organism capable of causing [the disease]''. These latter words, however, are omitted when section 35 is applied to AIDS by the 1988 Regulations.[57]

Further, section 35 envisages medical examination in the interests of the patient, his family or the public. Can it be justified in the interests of any of these to require a medical examination? In relation to the individual himself, the absence of an effective treatment or cure may call the scope of this provision into question. The availability of AZT may help to make the argument that it is in the patient's interests to know his HIV status but, of course, the Act does not deal with treatment itself. The public health goal in the AIDS epidemic has been to encourage voluntary testing and responsible behaviour thereafter, and so the application of section 35 to AIDS is, at best, surprising.

In relation to the interests of an individual's family, it has already been noted that their interests (e.g. of a sexual partner or spouse) may, as we have seen, justify, for instance, breaking confidence. Section 35 goes even further by countenancing the discovery of the information that a spouse or sexual partner might need in order to avoid the risk of transmission. But, of course, section 35 is not narrowly expressed in terms of there being a serious risk that infection may be transmitted, just in terms of the "interests of his family". Again the risk of transmission is less likely when the sexual partner is visibly ill— as he or she will be if they have developed AIDS—than in the case of the asymptomatic HIV infected partner. The logic of applying section 35 to AIDS in the way it has been is none too clear.

Removal to hospital: Section 37 authorises the removal of an AIDS sufferer (but not someone who is infected with HIV) to a hospital if:

1. proper precautions to prevent the spread of infection cannot be taken or are not being taken;
2. there is a serious risk of others being infected;
3. accommodation is available.

This section is potentially far-reaching in its impact on an individual's rights. However, since it is restricted to situations where a serious risk of infection arises because precautions cannot or are not being taken, it is limited in its effect. Rarely will such a situation arise because of the difficulty of transmitting the infection. It might, however, cover an AIDS patient who refuses to accept his doctor's advice to practise "safer sex" and thereby exposes his partner to the serious risk of infection. If this is the situation intended to be covered by section 37 it is curious that HIV positive individuals are not also covered because again it is here that the real risk (if any) could arise.

Detention in hospital: While section 37 only authorises removal to hospital, section 38 authorises detention for a period which must be specified in the court order but which may be subsequently extended. The Act gives no maximum period of detention. Section 38 (as modified by the Regulations[58]) permits detention if:

1. the person is suffering from AIDS,
2. is an in-patient in hospital,
3. on leaving hospital the individual *either* would not have suitable accommodation to allow proper precautions to be taken to prevent the spread of the disease *or* would not take proper precautions to prevent the spread of the disease at his accommodation or other places he might be expected to go.[59]

The power to detain for a finite period, but without limit on maximum length, is potentially a considerable restriction on an individual's rights. However, again section 38 (as modified) contains limitations. The section is clearly designed to prevent spread of the disease. It only applies when an individual is a danger to others. However, again, it only applies to AIDS and not HIV infection. Arguably, therefore, while significantly limiting freedom of movement, the provision misses its own public health goal.

The Government indicated when introducing the Regulations in 1985 that they were "intended for use in very exceptional circumstances".[60] Only one reported instance of their use exists, in Manchester in September 1985, when an order was made detaining an AIDS patient for three weeks. The order was subsequently lifted 10 days later by agreement after an appeal.[61] Nevertheless, the provisions of the Act represent a major challenge to individual rights on the basis of a concern for public health.

2. *Preferential discrimination*

Having reviewed areas of adverse discrimination, we should now explain the reference made earlier to preferential discrimination. Two examples are offered to illustrate the problem and to show how complex it is.

(a) Resource allocation in health care and generally It is undoubtedly true that the scale of the epidemic of HIV infection and AIDS means that ever greater demands will be placed on the health care system and on other social services (estimated at about £60 million extra over five years in 1988 for health care alone). The demands will be great because of the numbers involved, the length of time during which persons may be ill, the range of the illnesses involved and the consequent cost of caring for these illnesses. To take one example, if it be shown that if a person who is HIV positive but symptom-free takes certain drugs, he will postpone (or even, eventually prevent) the onset of AIDS the cost could be enormous. The target population is commonly young and the prophylaxis will be necessary for the rest of the person's life. Similarly, developments in the care of those with ARC or AIDS may prevent further deterioration or death but the patient may remain chronically ill, with consequent costs to health care and social services systems.

It is also true that many of those who have AIDS or are HIV positive have organised themselves into effective lobbies. The first aim of such lobbies has been to oppose and prevent adverse discrimination of the kinds which have been referred to. A second aim has been to maximise the care and support available. While this is entirely understandable, it poses a difficult problem of social policy. In most societies, planning the allocation of scarce health care resources is ultimately the task of governments. The issues involved are so complex, however, that planning often degenerates into reactive responses to pressure. Resources, human and material, are allocated where the pressure is greatest, often with short-term political goals in sight. A government does not wish to be thought to neglect new-born babies and so may allocate resources to neonatal intensive care units. But such an allocation has opportunity costs. There may be proportionately far more people who could benefit from mental health counselling or, in the case of the isolated elderly, domiciliary nursing. These may not be areas of dramatic life and death decisions, but, in health care terms they are of great importance. Equally, cervical cancer, which is eminently preventable, may continue to kill thousands of women annually through lack of screening facilities. Meanwhile, coronary care units blossom in a hundred hospitals (with doubtful results), since it is men who set the political agenda and men who have heart attacks! In short, planning gives way to lobbying and the loudest voice. Against such a background, the level of resources made available to those who are HIV positive or have AIDS will probably also be the product of pressure rather than rational calculation. A keen concern for human rights would suggest, however, that a society has an obligation to seek to ensure that others with other needs are not neglected or adversely discriminated against in the well-meaning desire to respond to the AIDS epidemic. It may well be an unpopular point to make. It may be that to make it is to run the risk of playing into the hands of those who favour discrimination against those with AIDS. It may be an enormously complex and ultimately insoluble conundrum. It should, however, be faced by a society committed to the protection and preservation of the human rights of all its citizens.

(b) Drug-testing and licensing The last year has seen decisions both in the US[62] and the UK to vary the normal practice which must be followed before drugs may lawfully be made available to patients on prescription. Ordinarily, there must be a lengthy process of carefully controlled trials. Licensing authorities (in effect the relevant government department) demand scrupulous evidence of safety, efficacy and quality before drugs are licensed. What has happened in the US is that, under pressure from a strong and articulate lobby, the licensing authorities have varied the procedure to be followed.[63] The effect of this is to permit drugs, thought as a consequence of preliminary research to be beneficial to patients with AIDS, to be made available to such patients in advance of confirmatory scientific trials. The argument in favour of this decision is superficially attractive. Patients are dying from an awful disease which appears to have a 100 per cent mortality. If a drug may have some beneficial effect, it can do no harm, it is said, to let these patients have it.

The counter-arguments may, however, be stronger. First, if it is thought that the only way to test drugs properly and establish their safety and efficacy is by the current methods of scientific trials, any departure from this approach either means that the drugs will (or may) not be safe or that the current method is unnecessary. Since the latter is not accepted, the former conclusion is inevitable. Secondly, the consequence of abandoning the traditional approach is that patients may receive drugs that may not only not benefit them but may indeed harm them. The harm may be either through unpredicted physical damage or through inducing them to rely on the particular drug (which is useless or harmful) and thereby to forgo other therapies which have been shown to be beneficial. Thirdly, the drugs involved may never be tested properly, because of the inability to carry out properly constituted trials, such that their validity can never be established. Fourthly, patients may find themselves manipulated by false reports and propaganda from drug companies and other vested interests (compare, for example, the advocacy of Laetrile in the US). The patients will as a consequence suffer while others, purporting to care for their interests, prosper.

The implications for human rights of these developments are real but complex.[64] It is rare that a commitment to human rights can take the form of an appeal to state paternalism. It may be, however, that this is an example where a society, to protect the vulnerable from themselves and from false hopes, should insist that drugs are not available until all normal scientific procedures have been satisfied. As a consequence, a society should resist any claim from a patient denied access to an as yet unlicensed drug that this constitutes a denial of human rights.[65]

Conclusion

Human rights, in the philosophical sense, have a significant role to play in developing good medical law. Nowhere is this more true than in the case of HIV infection and AIDS. Sufferers have much to benefit from an approach to their care which is informed by a concern for human rights. But will human rights law respond adequately? Clearly if it is to do so, it must be developed creatively. It must be seen as a dynamic force evolving as the real world which it seeks to regulate evolves. This development could come from the courts. The history of English law and to some extent of the European Court of Human Rights may leave us despairing at such a prospect. Certainly the law is there to be used in the form of the European Convention on Human Rights and Fundamental Freedoms. One need look no further than the masterly review written by the late Paul Sieghart shortly before his death in his *AIDS and Human Rights*.[66] Sieghart's approach was to identify first the policy options available to any state. These were, he suggested:

(a) *"Measures which can have no adverse effect on the human rights of any individuals."* Examples of these are, he suggested, research into the disease, ensuring the safety of blood for transfusion, preventing the re-use of needles and making safety devices such as condoms more freely available.

(b) *"Measures which could have an adverse effect, but which can only be implemented with the explicit, free and informed consent of the individual concerned."* Examples are voluntary testing for HIV infection, either on an "anonymous" basis, or with stringent safeguards, and counselling.

(c) *"Measures entailing compulsion."* Examples are mandatory screening of selected persons or groups, detention, quarantine, refusal of entry to a country, and exclusion from marriage, employment, housing, social services, or attendance at an educational institution.

Sieghart argues that such policies as are set out in (c), if contemplated, would have to be tested as regards their legitimacy by reference to whether they are "provided by law", are "necessary in a democratic society" and are for the protection of a legitimate aim which falls within a category in a relevant Article of the European Convention on Human Rights. His conclusion is that few would stand up to such scrutiny.

But if the courts, whether in the UK or Europe, do not act courageously then it must be the legislature which grasps the nettle. Some would argue that many of the issues are too controversial to encourage Parliamentary interest. Of course, there is something in this but controversy in itself is not an absolute ban on legislation even in the area of medicine and morals. The Human Fertilisation and Embryology Act 1990 pays tribute to that.

Issues of human rights and discrimination against HIV infected individuals and AIDS patients will not go away. Indeed they are likely to become more and more visible as the epidemic takes hold and threatens more. In this paper we have discussed only *some* of the important areas. Equally important are the problems of discrimination in education, in access to housing, and in prisons. Each of these situations frequently throws into conflict the interests and rights of the individual and others.

As regards education: how should a local education authority respond to parental protests if it is discovered that a teacher is HIV positive? Does a school have a right to know a child's HIV status? How should we respond to parents who refuse to allow their child to attend school where there is a child who is HIV positive? It is noteworthy that when the Government applied some of the provisions of the public health legislation to AIDS it specifically did not apply those parts which would prevent an infected child from attending school.

If we turn to consider prisons, is it consistent with the human rights of a prisoner to segregate him on the basis of his HIV status? Is it required out of respect for prisoners' rights to distribute condoms to prisoners to reduce the risk of transmitting the infection through the sexual contacts between prisoners whatever a narrow view of existing law may suggest?[67]

These and the other questions raised in this paper must be addressed as a matter of urgency. And they must be resolved in such a way that the commitment to human rights remains paramount.

Notes and references

1. Allen Lane, 1979.
2. See O'Brien, "Discrimination: the difference with AIDS" (1990) 6 *Journal of Contemporary Health Law and Policy* 93.
3. This has also been the World Health Organisation's global policy: see Mann, Dam and Kay, "Global coordination of national public health strategies" (1990) 18 *Law, Medicine and Health Care* 20.
4. Education was identified as the key component in any preventive programme in the *Harvard Model AIDS Legislative Project;* see Clark, "AIDS prevention: legislative options" (1990) 16 *American Journal of Law and Medicine* 107–55. See also Aiken, "Education as prevention", in Dalton and Burris eds, *AIDS and the Law* (1987) at 90.

5. For a masterly exposition of the issues see Sieghart, *AIDS and Human Rights: A UK Perspective* (British Medical Association, 1989).
6. Statement of General Medical Council, "HIV Infection and AIDS: The Ethical Considerations", paragraph 7 (May 1988).
7. Ibid.
8. See *Guidance for Clinical Health Care Workers: Protection Against Infection with HIV and Hepatitis Viruses* (HMSO, January 1990).
8a. But see now the case of the Florida dentist, at least four of whose patients were infected by him. Precisely how they came to be infected may never be known.
9. See *AIDS: HIV-Infected Health Care Workers* (HMSO, March 1988) for proper precautionary measures.
10. The most thorough and scholarly analysis of the public policy issues can be found in Field, "Testing for AIDS: uses and abuses" (1990) 16 *American Journal of Law and Medicine* 33–107. See also Hodgson, "The legal and public policy implications of human immunodeficiency virus antibody testing in New Zealand", in *Legal Implications of AIDS* (Legal Research Foundation, Auckland, 1989) at 39–95.
11. Statement of General Medical Council, "HIV Infection and AIDS: The Ethical Considerations", paragraphs 12–14.
12. Ibid. at paragraph 13.
13. See Kennedy and Grubb, "The legality of testing for HIV infection (1989) 86 *Law Society Gazette* (7) at 32 and (9) at 30. See also A. Grubb and D. Pearl, *Blood Testing, Aids and DNA Profiling: Law and Policy* (Jordans, 1990) chapter 1.
14. This is not to say that controversy does not exist over the need for explicit consent. See the discussion in Keown, "The ashes of AIDS and the phoenix of informed consent" (1989) 52 *Modern Law Review* 790 who, in his conclusions, arguably underestimates the potential for dynamic development of the common law by the judiciary.
15. For a description of the scheme see, *HIV and AIDS* (1990), at 40 (Virginia Bottomly MP).
16. For an argued case in favour of anonymised testing see Field, op. cit. at 51–53 suggesting that the provision of anonymised testing may encourage others to seek voluntary testing.
17. See Kennedy and Grubb op. cit.
18. Sex Discrimination Act 1975.
19. Race Relations Act 1976.
20. The case is discussed in *AIDS: A Guide to the Law* (Terrence Higgins Trust, 1990) at 93–4.
21. Napier, "AIDS, discrimination and employment law" (1989) 18 *Industrial Law Journal* 84, 87.
22. Napier op. cit. at 88.
23. [1987] ICR 700,000 per Dillon LJ.
24. See e.g. *Cormack v. TNT Sealion Ltd* (1986) (unreported).

25. See *Buck* v. *The Letchworth Palace Ltd* (1986) (unreported).
26. Napier, op. cit. at 94.
27. Napier, op. cit. at 95.
28. See *AIDS: A Guide to the Law* op. cit. appendix 3.
29. For a clear discussion of the issues see Scherzer, in *AIDS and the Law* op. cit. at 185.
30. e.g. *Rozanes* v. *Bowen* (1928) 32 Lloyd's Law Reports 98. See also, *London Assurance* v. *Mansel* (1879) 11 Ch D 363.
31. [1908] 2 KB 863,884.
32. See *Ionides* v. *Pender* (1874) LR 9 QB 531. But note the alternative test looking at it from the assured's point of view in *Joel* v. *Law Union Assurance Co* [1908] 2 KB 863, 883–4 per Fletcher Moulton LJ.
33. The contract of insurance would be *voidable* by the insurance company. See, for example, *Mackender* v. *Felida AG* [1966] 2 Lloyd's Reports 449,455 per Lord Denning MR.
34. See 7th Report (1588–9), *AIDS*, HC 202, para 18.
35. See Clifford and Iuculano, "AIDS and insurance: the rationale for AIDS-related testing" (1987) 100 *Harvard Law Review* 1806.
36. See Access to Medical Reports Act 1988.
37. Set out in Edgar and Sandomire, "Medical privacy issues in the age of AIDS: legislative options" (1990) 16 *American Journal of Law and Medicine* 155 at 215–19.
38. The public policy arguments are examined in Edgar and Sandomire, "Medical privacy issues in the age of AIDS: legislative options" (1990) 16 *American Journal of Law and Medicine* 155–222.
39. For a discussion see A. Grubb and D. Pearl, op. cit. chapter 2.
40. See Kennedy and Grubb, *Medical Law: Text and Materials* (Butterworths, 1989) at 160–7.
41. For example, *X* v. *Y* [1988] 2 All ER 648 and *W* v. *Edgell* [1990] 1 All ER 835.
42. SI 1974/29. Discussed in A. Grubb and D. Pearl, op. cit. at 39–41.
43. [1988] 2 All ER 648 at 653 per Rose J.
44. See A. Grubb and D. Pearl, op. cit. at 42–57 and *W* v. *Edgell* [1990] 1 All ER 835 at 848–9 per Bingham LJ (giving examples where disclosure might be justified).
45. See Grubb and Pearl, op. cit. at 55–6.
46. See *GMC Statement*.
47. See *Guidance for Clinical Health Care Workers* (HMSO, 1990) op. cit.
48. See *GMC Statement* paragraph 19.
49. Grubb and Pearl, op. cit. at 43–8.
50. Grubb and Pearl, op. cit. at 48–55.
51. See Edgar and Sandomire, op. cit.; disclosure to crime victims (at 194–6); in prisons and mental institutions (at 196–9); to school authorities (at 199–201); to funeral directors (at 201–2); to protect the blood supply (at 202–3); in cases of tissue or organ donation (at 203–4).
52. It was this policy which led many including the British Government

to boycott the 1990 World AIDS Conference held in San Francisco.
53. WHO/SPA/GLO/87.1.
54. Paragraph 4.
55. Public Health (Infectious Diseases) Regulations 1985 (SI 1985/434). See now Public Health (Infectious Diseases) Regulations 1988 (SI 1988/1546).
56. The 1988 Regulations (ibid.) extend various of the provisions of the Act to a whole range of other diseases; see schedule 1.
57. See Regulation 4.
58. Regulation 5.
59. It is this latter addition of "other places to which [the patient] might be expected to go . . ." which is added by Regulation 5.
60. HC 1341, para 593. See the discussion in Grubb and Pearl, "English law and issues relating to medicine, health and the family", in Banakas ed., *United Kingdom Law in the 1980s*, (UKN CCL) 120 at 123–5.
61. Discussed ibid.
62. Discussed in Cooper, "Changes in normal drug approval process in response to the AIDS crisis" (1990) 45 *Food Drug and Cosmetic Law Journal* 329.
63. The arguments of one AIDS activist are stated in Eigo, "Expedited drug approval procedures: perspectives from an AIDS activist" (1990) 45 *Food Drug and Cosmetic Law Journal* 377.
64. The legal issues are discussed in Kiser, "Legal issues raised by expedited approval of, and expanded access to, experimental AIDS treatments" (1990) 45 *Food Drug and Cosmetic Law Journal* 363.
65. See the discussion by George Annas, "FDA's compassion for desperate drug companies" (1990) *Hastings Center Report* (number 1) 35.
66. British Medical Association, 1989.
67. Current policy is to oppose the distribution of condoms because it would require Government to connive in the commission of a crime. It is a crime for a man to engage in homosexual conduct with another in a public place. Prisons, it is agreed, are public places.

Ethics and regulation in randomised controlled trials of therapy

Gayle Rawlings

Introduction

Interest in the underlying ethical principles and regulations of health care has been growing dramatically since World War II, with a particularly rapid increase in the last decade. Many reasons for this come to mind, but they all seem to share a common underpinning. Members of the health care and legal professions, as well as governments, philosophers, sociologists, economists, and the general public, have become acutely aware of the fact that all medical actions have consequences which extend much further than the effects noted in individual patients. At the same time, the way we conceptualise medical care has been changing; we no longer see the patient only as a passive recipient of a medical intervention, but also as a client–partner in a mutual enterprise of seemingly ever-expanding scope. Thus, our decisions about which rights we will ascribe to the patient-client, and which duties we feel the role of physician demands, must always be made in view of the two contexts. At the same time as attempting to establish the optimal legal and ethical framework for the individual doctor–patient relationship, we must also be aware of the possible impact of that choice of framework on wider society. Whether or not our moral decisions are based on consequences alone, it is rare indeed to find arguments that they should be disregarded altogether. Now, in the context of late 20th century medical practice, we find the question, *"whose* consequences matter?" being posed with ever greater urgency alongside the traditional one, "how much weight should consequences have?" There is obviously much potential for viewing health care today as inevitably containing an "individual versus society" conflict, and the literature in this area amply illustrates this.

Nowhere is this seen more vividly than in discussions of the morality of human experimentation. Here there is no shortage of debate, representing all points of view, from enthusiastic acceptance to categorical rejection. In this paper, I will confine myself to consideration of one subset of clinical research, the randomised controlled trial; and I will be making particular reference to its use in the assessment of forms of treatment of cancer. Even within this restricted field, the same wide range of opinions on its ethical permissibility exists. That consensus seems so far off among those who clearly share a profound concern for human welfare, makes it all the more necessary that differing stances be considered carefully, and the supporting principles be clearly understood and weighed. In doing so, even though I will deal with only a small area of medicine, many of the difficult problems in health care will be illuminated.

In order to explore the need for, and justification of, clinical trials, it is necessary to take a step backward to look at how current medical practitioners have come by their "knowledge".

The type of education which transforms a (generally) young, idealistic, enthusiastic layperson into a licensed physician has traditionally emphasised the acquisition of verifiable facts and the attainment of useful skills. First year medical students sweating to memorise intricate details of cardiac physiology have little inclination and even less time to reflect on the professional and ethical battles fought to bring this knowledge to light. These students are only separated by a few centuries from their counterparts, who learned as dogma Galen's textbook diagrams of human anatomy (later shown to be total fabrications or based on pigs); ethical and religious prohibition of the use of human cadavers for dissection and teaching was the norm as late as 16th century Europe, where Andreas Vesalius scandalised the establishment by stealing the bodies of hanged men off the gallows for his studies. Students in the 1980s, however, would consider (should they think of such things at all) that the gulf separating them from these quaint figures is one not only of time, but more importantly, of a diametrically different approach to medical knowledge. They would argue that their rapidly growing fund of useful facts was obtained through a scientific method which demands objective verification and encourages further investigation, rather than by tradition or belief; and they would feel themselves to be free of moral conflict in their pursuit of those facts and skills which will enable them to practise medicine well.

How accurate are these students in their assessment of the current state of affairs? In my view, they are allowing a small portion of truth to obscure a great deal of illusion. True, scientific method did produce *part* of the data base they are mastering; but it was someone else's scientific method, testing of hypotheses, nights of doubt which achieved it. No medical curriculum has the luxury of enough time to allow painstaking rediscovery of information now considered standard; the unfortunate result is that medical students must absorb more ''received truth'' than in any theological discipline, and tend to feel comfortable with it as a result. This leads to a tendency to blur together those ''facts'' whose ''veracity'' derives from scientific testing with ''facts'' accepted because of tradition, theoretical worth, or biased observation. And it is not surprising that this is the case. In medical school and most specialty programmes, it is the current body of accepted knowledge that is examined, not the way in which it came to be accepted. It is the hard truth that it is in the part of medicine where physicians have the most impact on their patients, in therapeutic manoeuvres, that they have the least proof of the value of what they do. Doctors must, in general, offer treatment with an inadequate understanding of its effect on the patient, and without reliable reasons for favouring it over different courses of action. This creates difficulties enough, but they are compounded when medical education encourages practitioners to feel secure and confident in the therapeutics they have mastered, rather than acutely aware of the limitations of their knowledge.

Less ethical or scientific debate attaches to the skills associated with diagnosis and the implementation of designated therapy, such as the mastery of electrocardiogram interpretation or chest X-ray analysis, or the performance of the removal of a gall bladder. The extrapolation of these skills to the real world raises many moral questions. How much should patients be inconvenienced in order to permit medical students to learn how to interview and examine them? What risks are permissible when students learn invasive procedures, even under supervision? The application of even the least controversial of facts can lead to disturbing ethical dilemmas. The patient, the doctor, and all of society have expectations of health care, and potentially differing views of what would constitute the ideal. Because the purpose of any form of medical experimentation is to improve the provision of health care (given that the perfect world where it is no longer necessary seems permanently unattainable), it is essential to examine the notion of the ideal in health care, before entering into the specifics of clinical trials research. The scenario proposed is at a practical level, and is based around the illness- or problem-oriented medical model. This is not to deny the importance of preventative medicine and health education, merely to narrow the focus here to that part of health care with direct relevance to the controlled comparisons of therapy which will subsequently be discussed. The analysis will also be restricted to the competent adult patient.

In this scenario we would have the following:

An individual with a problem consults a physician: Skilful interviewing, examination, and selection of appropriate tests lead to rapid and accurate diagnosis of the problem.

The physician recommends a course of action: Tradition, historical experience, pharmacological study and animal experiments will have suggested certain approaches; their comparative worth will have been verified clinically by the appropriate human trials; and the physician will be aware of the results through education, publication and conferences, and thus be able to judge what to recommend to the patient, and to accurately describe the alternatives.

The patient decides: Full, honest, and reliable information, given in the context of a relationship of trust and confidence, allow the patient to choose the most personally suitable treatment plan.

The plan is implemented: An educated, motivated, cooperative health care team work with the patient to carry out what has been decided; funds and facilities are available to do this in the way intended.

It can readily be appreciated that we have a long way to go, to achieve this ideal in the 1990s. In many, if not most, areas of medicine there is no one best course of action. All current approaches may be deemed unacceptable, or there may be multiple "equally good" choices, of more or less usefulness.

What is much more vexing, and gives rise to the profoundly difficult questions of human experimentation, is that the validity of most recommended approaches is in dispute. Personal anecdotal experience, published historical results, conjecture based on results in animals or possibly comparable diseases, are the usual reasons for outlining a certain treatment plan (as well, as was discussed earlier, an unquestioning belief in what was taught in medical school or residency); these justifications for therapeutic decisions are grossly inadequate to assess the worth of manoeuvres which will have such impact on human lives.

Beyond this, even if what is "best" therapy has been conclusively demonstrated, we have to look closely at which endpoints are used to arrive at this conclusion. A treatment which leads to the highest cure rates may also have unavoidable or potential harmful effects which a less effective remedy avoids. And, even if an intervention would be considered "best" on all grounds (i.e. easiest to tolerate, best cure rate, fewest side-effects, least expensive) it is by no means certain that the individual practitioner has even heard about it, or if so, believes it. Many well designed and convincing clinical trials have had limited impact as their results were not publicised adequately to the relevant part of the medical community. And further, what is recommended may be refused for many reasons other than the patient's honest awareness of having different needs and values to those of the doctor's. Fear, ignorance, prejudice, poor rapport, and simple misunderstanding all play a large role in the step between the offer and the acceptance of treatment.

Finally, even if the chain of events could take place without mishap to this point, an ever increasing problem looms. We may not be able to carry out this recommended and accepted proven best course of action, due to inadequate equipment, lack of support staff, poor medical skills, problems of cooperation with other medical specialties, and a shortage of funds. What the medical profession recommends and what the government pays for are two different things; this facet of tax-supported health care makes it all the more crucial that what is advocated has been scientifically validated.

The world we live in continually falls short of the ideal, and the attainment of a medical model such as that proposed remains far off. Even if all current difficulties with methodology, accrual, and ethics in clinical trials were solved instantly, multiple problems in health care delivery would persist. Conversely, however, without a valid means to assess the worth of prescribed treatment, the remainder of medical practice rests on an extremely unstable foundation.

All of the above becomes particularly acute where cancer therapy is considered. For most adult cancers, cure rates are poor, and side-effects and complications of treatment remain common and are frequently devastating. Subspecialty bias influences most recommendations, and cooperation between specialists is frequently grudging. Nowhere is the need for testing of current and new approaches more readily demonstrable. How can this be accomplished, and what human costs are involved?

Controlled clinical trials

Clinical trials are largely a post World War II phenomenon. In part, this was due to the war itself; Rothman[1] argues convincingly that the sacrifices made by conscripts and volunteers in battle led to increasing willingness to involve human beings in experimentation to assess risks and therapies of many diseases, largely communicable or tropical. In addition, the development of expensive antibiotics, in such short supply that few patients could receive them, meant that controlled studies of their effectiveness were imperative. The statistical methodology for assessing such investigation had become sufficiently advanced, and acceptance in the scientific community of its worth was beginning to be possible. As late as the 19th century, however, considerable debate raged over whether by studying groups of patients one could draw conclusions relevant to individual cases. Armitage[2] quotes a debate between F. J. Double and Pierre Louis in Paris in 1835:

Double states: "For myself I must say that the more I see of a disease the more does each case appear to me a new and a separate problem . . . Individuality is an invariant element in pathology . . . Numerical and statistical calculations, open to many sources of fallacy, are in no degree applicable to therapeutics."

Louis responds: "A therapeutic agent cannot be employed with any discrimination or probability of success in a given case, unless its general efficacy, in analogous cases, has been previously ascertained; therefore I conceive that without the aid of statistics nothing like real medical science is possible."

Although the latter view is now generally accepted, the importance of individuality is not overlooked, but taken into account in trials design. Indeed, its influence is one of the major factors mandating for randomisation in such studies.

When we consider the special case of cancer treatment, we also find in the post-war years the development of major Cancer Centres in North America, the UK, and Europe. These, plus the establishment or rapid growth of important sources of funding for basic and clinical research (e.g. the Medical Research Council in the UK, or President Nixon's "War on Cancer" in the US), have provided the impetus for concerned clinician-investigators to initiate large-scale intervention trials.

Why has it come to be accepted that the randomised controlled clinical trial (or RCT) is by far the most reliable form of clinical investigation? An examination of the problems associated with drawing conclusions from other types of study is illuminating.

It simply is not possible to learn enough about the effects of treatment on human beings from animal experimentation. The ethical problems associated with potentially harmful and painful experimentation on sentient living beings who cannot consent are not negligible. Even assuming that they could be satisfactorily resolved, safety and effectiveness in animals is never an invariable predictor of the same result in humans. Moreover, many disease states, including most types of cancer, simply cannot be found (or caused) in animals.

What then can be learned from careful examination of the outcome of treatment given to an individual patient? Any form of therapy is, after all, an interventional trial, a form of human experimentation—in which an attempt is made to prove the hypothesis that of all the types of treatment the doctor has considered, the recommended one is likeliest to lead to the desired result for this patient. What must be acknowledged, however, is that all we can ever learn from this use of therapy is whether the intervention was *followed by* the desired outcome. Whether good results occurred because of, independent of, or in spite of the treatment cannot be determined. The fallacy of *post hoc propter hoc* reasoning has been part of medical practice since its first history, and continues to this day.

Doctors have also attempted to assess the effect of therapy by means of pilot studies, where a number of patients are given the same treatment, generally new and felt to be promising. As Pocock[3] and many others have pointed out, the history of modern medicine is replete with apparent advances which enthusiastic practitioners have sincerely believed to be real (and cancer treatment is no exception). Unfortunately, as often as not, later evaluation by RCT shows them to be no better, and often worse, than the standard therapy they were meant to replace. Silverman[4] illustrates this graphically. There are many possible reasons why these treatments which offer no improvement are initially thought to. There is no discounting the power of the placebo effect. Any medical intervention, particularly one in which the doctor has great confidence, can lead to increased patient wellbeing, even without this improvement being a result of the therapy. Also, selection bias may play a part, with the patients who are offered the "improved" therapy being the ones with the greatest chance of cure in any case. And finally, as Engelhardt[5] comments, the psychology of discovery leads clinicians to be biased in favour of seeing the world as they expect, or feel it ought to be. Erroneous interpretation of data, and unconscious slanting of the perception of the worth of clinical interventions, is continually going on. It is not easily seen by investigators or their contemporaries, for the obvious reason that their biases prevent this: but we are readily able to see it in the judgments of previous decades, and the failures to corroborate pilot studies give us good reasons to assume it persists.

Prospective studies using historical controls have also been frequently used. In them, the results of test therapy are compared with those obtained with standard therapy in previous patients. If one could be certain that the current test group of patients are identical to the historical controls in every way, this would be a scientifically valid assessment; there are many reasons why this is rarely the case. These include differences in patient selection, poor quality of recorded data in the historical group, differences in evaluating response, improved ancillary care for the later group of patients, and the tendency to invalidate current patients faring badly initially on the new treatment. It is therefore common for trials using historical controls to exaggerate the benefit of the new treatment, or to claim one where none exists. Prospective studies using concurrent controls are therefore much to be preferred, but if the choice of assignment of therapy is left to the investigator or patient, or is predictable in any way, selection bias remains a huge stumbling-block to the validity of the apparent results. If there is any difference between the two groups of patients, other than the treatment they have received, our ability to be sure that any difference in outcome is in fact due to the treatment is diminished considerably.

All this being said, it should be noted that a huge improvement in treatment would not require a randomised clinical trial to be accepted. Where a previously inevitably fatal illness is found to be cured 90 per cent of the time by a new combination of drugs, one feels confident that historical controls are sufficient. Realistically, however, such large differences in apparent cure rates are all too rare, and the modest gains that proposed new therapies might cause are generally in the order of only 10 to 20 per cent. Such improvements could only be reliably established by RCT; but for the common malignancies such as lung, bowel, and breast cancer, even a 10 per cent increase in cure rate translates into thousands of lives saved from a premature and painful end. Furthermore, an equally important use of RCT methodology is to establish that two different therapies have no difference in their cure rates. (Attempts to demonstrate that less mutilating surgery leads to cure rates equivalent to that achieved with radical procedures would fall into this category.) The biases inherent in uncontrolled, historical, or unrandomised studies mean that they will not, and should not, convince most members of the medical community of the equivalence of treatments.

The RCT, then, is a form of therapeutic investigation which, (1) compares a control group (patients treated in currently standard fashion, or with placebo if no effective treatment exists) with a group receiving an experimental therapy, or an alternative standard one; and (2) compares groups formed by random assignment such that neither the patient nor the investigator influences the choice of treatment.

The whole reason for doing trials of the effectiveness of treatment is to allow doctors to offer interventions with the chance of doing the most good for the patient. It is worse than useless to perform "trials of therapy" where many other factors than the therapy itself bear on the outcome. Random assignment is the best way of avoiding this, but the methodology of carrying out these trials is complex, and there are many practical problems.

I do not wish to dwell on these technical aspects, except to note that studies which are badly designed, executed, or analysed (and such studies are unfortunately not rare) can only lead to unpublishable or misleading results. Just as the unskilful setting of a fractured bone can leave the patient worse off than before, similarly a poorly executed RCT wastes the opportunity to learn anything and the efforts of the patients and investigators participating in it.

It also cannot be stated strongly enough that the amount of hard work and dedication involved in organising RCTs is immense. Additional personnel, rooms, facilities will be needed, all of which must be paid for; meetings with other parties involved, such as pharmaceutical companies, must be arranged; additional training for nurses, radiotherapy technicians, and other health care workers involved must be provided; other doctors or institutes must be coordinated with; and ongoing monitoring of the intervention to assure uniformity and quality control must be instituted. So even before we begin to explore the ethical problems RCTs may give rise to, it is clear that in any case they are difficult, time-consuming, and frustrating enterprises in the best of circumstances (i.e. when the respect of one's colleagues and ascent of the academic ladder may result from organising or participating in them); the financial reward is always greater in a non-research, standard clinical practice, and is much greater in countries where private practice is permitted. In most areas of medicine, RCTs are not proposed, or fail to attract enough support from the doctors to get underway. Although some do argue that trials are unnecessary, more commonly the view is expressed, in published reports of uncontrolled experiments, that the definitive answer to whether the described treatment is an improvement requires a randomised controlled trial. This lip service does not often lead to such a trial being performed, however, and well-intentioned unvalidated interventions may be adopted, causing patients needless harm. Or, conversely, changes in therapy which are truly of benefit will not be offered, as clinicians have no way to be sure of their worth and will not risk harm without it.

Ethical problems

There is a strong argument that it is not only permissible, but imperative for RCTs to be performed. It takes its force from two strong positions. The first, a consequentialist one, looks at the result of *not* doing RCTs. It sees future patients, or in other words all of society, as being harmed by the continuation of ineffective and harmful practices which would otherwise have been avoided, as well as missing out on the benefit of innovations which could have been shown to be effective. The truth of this cannot be disputed and to those whose only concern is the crude utilitarian "greatest good for the greatest number" there can be no question that well-designed and well-executed RCTs to answer crucial questions in treatment must be performed. Even for those whose moral judgments include consideration of rights, duties, and interests, the great harm that will result if such research is not done is a powerful factor, although not by itself a deciding one.

To arrive at the second reason why RCTs are ethically imperative, one must start off by asking if medical care *per se* is only an optional good. The fact that fee-paying patients solicit it would not by itself show that society feels it necessary; but as taxpayers are willing to support it, not just for their own families but for everyone, and we talk of the *right* to health care, it is safe to say that, in the UK at least, medical care is not considered a privilege, but a moral necessity. It then should follow that the delivery of this care in such a way as to lead to better understanding of what will be effective and safe is equally a necessity and should be demanded by society of itself. Such an argument of course is irrelevant to non-therapeutic human experimentation; but where a patient needs and has the right to treatment in any case, then providing it in such a way as to guide future medical approaches must be equally imperative. Here, as well, we can agree with the argument, all else being equal; but we must now look carefully at some reasons why all else may not be equal in clinical trials research. I will examine them in three broad categories: problems with human experimentation *per se,* problems related to consent, and problems inherent in RCT design.

Human experimentation

We should first deal with a problem which is generally considered to be one of ethics, but which properly falls within the category of an emotional or psychological objection. Any research proposal which involves human beings, whether or not it is a trial of therapy, evokes the "gut" reaction that they are being merely used, like guinea pigs or things, rather than being regarded in their full humanity as ends in themselves. We are not far enough away from the horrors of sadistic experimentation in Nazi Germany to be able to think dispassionately about what is involved, and perhaps this is all to the good. It is infinitely to be preferred that all human experimentation be viewed with suspicion, and as a course of last resort, than that it be accepted unquestioningly. It is true that people are used merely as a means if they are not informed that they are subjects of research, or if deceit is used to get their participation. But in the specific instance of clinical comparisons of therapy, patients are indeed regarded and treated as ends in themselves, in addition to knowingly being used as means to an important end *which they themselves share,* namely the improvement of medical care for all. Jonas[6], one of the most eloquent proponents of the view that experimentation is dehumanising, writes, "What is wrong with making a person an experimental subject is . . . that we make him a thing—a passive thing, merely to be acted upon." It is very difficult to find his philosophical basis for maintaining that even with consent, the research subject is *merely* being acted upon. In any case, he makes it clear that his arguments only apply to non-therapeutic research. He would be willing to accept as ethical the consenting participation of even a dying patient (i.e. one who could not possibly benefit) in research on his own disease, because the patient would identify with the aims of the research. Sharing in the ends of the experiment, even if there is no hope of personal benefit, is thus seen by him as a good which removes the passivity and dehumanising aspects of research; many who quote his arguments fail to note this. If, then, the Kantian imperative of never using persons merely as means is respected here, then our shrinking from RCTs, merely because they are a form of research, is not based on a violation of ethical principle, but on an emotional wish *not to be used at all*—an understandable desire. Since it is a desire which is never fulfilled in ordinary medical care, nor in most activities of life, it does not seem an adequate reason to refrain from clinical research. However, other cogent arguments are advanced for rejecting any form of research trials on humans. The problems of scientific priority and the pressures this inevitably places on the clinician-researcher are increasingly prominent. It is true that the present climate of demand for multiple publications, within some areas of academic medicine, has encouraged the rapid development of protocols to test new drugs and therapeutic manoeuvres. There is a danger that this academic and peer pressure may adversely colour researchers' attitudes toward permissible patient risks and need for real consent. This theoretical risk to research is not one which in my view should constitute a barrier to research, but could act as a stimulus to ensuring that it is performed in the most ethically appropriate manner. Those same pressures of peer review can be used to encourage the maintenance of the principles of respect for persons and avoiding harm; this opportunity for exposing ethical concerns in treatment is an advantage that is not available to the patient who is treated in standard fashion by a relatively isolated practitioner.

Another objection, brought forward by Giertz,[7] is the possible adverse effect of the RCT on the doctor–patient relationship. This concern is shared by many members of the medical profession, and an influential study reported by Taylor *et al.*,[8] on problems of accrual for an international breast cancer study, cited physician worries about the doctor–patient relationship to be a factor for 73 per cent of surgeons who did not enrol all eligible patients. In the desire to do no harm to their patients, many doctors who are persuaded that such a disruption in physician-patient relationship is inevitable, have declined to offer their patients participation in research; other doctors, equally persuaded that knowledge of trial participation will disrupt their relationships with patients, have argued instead that such patients should not be informed that they are part of an experiment. They are convinced that the possible good of such research mitigates its performance under such less-than-honest circumstances.

Do we have information which will allow us to decide if performing RCTs does in fact harm the bond of trust and mutual respect which is the ideal of medical practice? Cassileth *et al.*[9] surveyed members of the general public, cardiac patients, and cancer patients (all in the US), for their attitudes toward research on human beings, and found that the majority felt that clinical research was important, ethical and consistent with best medical treatment. Kemp[10] conducted interview surveys of 1022 adult members of the general public in the UK, with the express purpose of canvassing attitudes toward participating in clinical trials, but secondarily determining levels of information patients wished from their doctors, and how this influenced their confidence in them. A very strong response in favour of RCTs, and of patients being given full information, was obtained. In this study of non-patients, a high level of confidence in doctors was demonstrated, and it was not diminished by the recommendation of enrolment in controlled research. Thus, the paternalistic attitude of the medical profession towards patients' willingness to accept altruistic research is thrown into question. Much more remains to be learned about the ideal ways for care-givers and patients to relate; currently it seems reasonable to assume that soliciting patient participation in a well-designed trial, which the physician can support confidently, need not worsen the therapeutic interaction, and may in fact strengthen it.

Consent

More attention is focused on difficulties with consent than any other area of RCTs. An initial set of objections has to do with the harm attempting to obtain it can cause, and the correlated position that obtaining is not necessary. Brewin[11] espouses a belief that was common in North America until the 1970s, and which still has adherents in the UK. He argues that in therapeutic research, where the patient requires (and the clinician wishes to give) the best possible form of treatment, any research project which is ethical does not require special consent, over and above that required for any form of treatment. If a physician can honestly recommend participation in a trial, it can only be because of confidence that no difference in results is known and that the patient will be receiving the optimal form of therapy in any case. He therefore considers it an intrusion to inform the patient that such therapy is assigned by randomisation in an experiment. Other disadvantages he cites to the practice of requiring full consent are the anxiety it gives rise to (particularly in the UK where, apart from surgical procedures, written consent is rarely requested), and the perception he has that patients would prefer not to know all about their treatment and its possible outcome.

It is possible to refute his arguments about the possible harm that requiring consent can lead to. The experience previously noted of Kemp,[12] where desire for full disclosure was very common, points to the advantages for patient rapport when full information is forthcoming. Penman et al.[13] describe a New York experience, where fully informed consent for investigational chemotherapy was routinely solicited, and over 80 per cent of the patients interviewed felt that the amount of information they were given was "just right". It has been a constant feature of the medical profession's paternalistic stance that harm is a frequent result of disclosure; the absence of tangible evidence to this effect, and continuing information suggesting otherwise, make this a difficult position to maintain.

And if it could be shown that some patients might be harmed by the information required for valid consent to being a trial participant, there is still no reason to argue that this justifies enrolling them without their knowledge. It points strongly to the reverse, that they should not be considered for an RCT at all. The position that fully informed, uncoerced consent is vital to the morality of any research involving the treatment of human beings derives from the principle that in any situation where people risk harm, or may be deprived of a possible benefit, they are not being respected as ends in themselves if they have not been able to choose or refuse that situation. That they are being treated merely as a means, if not allowed to make their own, autonomous choice, is independent of whether harm or benefit in fact results. Such a position would argue that no one has an obligation or duty to enter into therapeutic research, that it can only be conducted on a volunteer basis. Caplan[14] interestingly asserts the viewpoint that although abstract duties to society cannot be demonstrated, there are specific ways in which those who accept the benefits of social cooperation (such as treatment in publicly funded research-oriented cancer institutes) are bound by principles of fair play to participate in research. The argument could then be extended against the need for consent, as one does not need to volunteer to do one's duty. The principle of justice could also be invoked, but to refute this argument. It cannot be fair that people, already burdened with a potentially fatal disease, should in some circumstances not be given the option of participation or refusal in research, merely on the basis of a referral pattern usually outside their control. It is not the potential risk to the patient of becoming a study subject, but the principle of respect for persons, which requires that they be true volunteers.

This leads directly to a challenging argument: are those who give their consent to participation in trials really acting as volunteers? Fully informed consent, which is essential to volunteering, may not be harmful, and should not be optional, but in the final analysis may simply be impossible. The patients agreeing to receiving their treatment as part of a trial may be doing so without adequate understanding, and may have been subject to a subtle form of coercion.

In the Penman study previously quoted, the primary reason for giving consent was "trust in the physician", and for the majority "the information given per se was not the prime determinant in reaching a positive decision" (to participate in the study). Cassileth and co-workers[15] interviewed cancer patients the day after written informed consent to treatment was obtained, and reported major deficits: 40 per cent did not understand the nature and purpose of the treatment, only 45 per cent could give even one major risk or complication, and only 40 per cent read the consent form carefully. Although improvements have been made in the techniques and reliability of informed consent, it remains true that patients who are considering entry into a trial are bound to be influenced by the understandable desire to please the person responsible for their care, and by their trust in that person; their own understanding of the information presented, and their personal treatment preferences, may be given less weight than is consistent with an autonomous, uncoerced choice.

But even here, strong counter-arguments can be brought. When a UK comparative trial of mastectomy versus conservative breast surgery was attempting to enlist patient participation, full information about the options led to widespread refusal to enter the trial. In this circumstance, patients obviously were adequately informed about alternatives, and far from feeling coerced, decided on the basis of personal preference that a random assignment to one or other treatment was unacceptable. A similar pattern of patient refusal occurred in the US and Canada with an NSABP (National Surgical Adjuvant Breast and Bowel Project) trial of breast cancer treatment, and has been noticed as well in studies of therapy in patients with metastatic prostate cancer. One of the reasons why investigators find informed consent requirements a hindrance to accrual is that patients with strong enough personal preferences do *not* hesitate to use them as a reason to decline study participation; those refusals are a hopeful sign that respect for persons and the preservation of the right to autonomous choice can be, and are, features of RCTs.

And even if truly informed, uncoerced consent to research participation is more difficult to be sure of than we are aware, surely this is even more true of the "standard therapy" which will be given if no trial is conducted. The vulnerability of patients, particularly in their dependent role on physicians, makes the preservation of their status as individuals with dignity and autonomy a continuing priority in all parts of medicine, not just research to evaluate treatment. That we as a society have not perfected this preservation yet does not deter us from caring for the sick as an ethical good; why then (so long as there are continuing efforts to achieve it) should it prevent the acceptance of otherwise ethically acceptable research?

A final, utilitarian objection to the obtaining of informed consent is often made, namely that more patients will participate, a more representative sample of patients will be studied, and trials will be completed faster (thus other patients will benefit sooner), if it is unnecessary. While the truth of this assertion cannot be disputed in some circumstances, local custom and prevailing fashion may be the main reason for it. In the largest cancer treatment centre in Canada, the Princess Margaret Hospital in Toronto, written informed consent to enrolment in RCTs became a requirement in the 1970s. Initially, accrual rates were unexpectedly low in some trials, both for reasons of patient refusal, and of physician unwillingness to go through the (then thought to be) arduous process of soliciting consent. As the general public in Canada has become more familiar with the concept of the randomised trial, and doctors more comfortable with discussing their uncertainty about best treatment, i.e.

admitting medical fallibility, the acceptance rates for most trials, even very complex ones, have greatly improved. While more research into reasons why patients refuse trials is needed, and such studies are currently being undertaken by Sutherland and co-workers in Toronto[16], it is not necessarily true that patient refusal need remain a stumbling block to obtaining adequate and representative participation in RCTs; but if respect for patient autonomy is paramount, informed refusals are inevitable and an important check on medical practice.

Randomised controlled trial design

The accuracy of the information which can be obtained from a comparative trial of therapy is dependent on the equivalence of the groups being analysed, apart from the treatment received. Random assignment is necessary to ensure this, but ethical objections to assigning treatment on a random basis are frequently raised.

One potential problem is the risk of harm to those patients who do not receive the treatment ultimately shown to be the most beneficial. This risk is often believed to be higher than the risks any patient must face when being treated in currently standard fashion, not in an RCT. Although this objection to randomisation seems to have merit, and there must be good reasons and supporting evidence for proposing a trial of a new form of therapy, proof of its superiority is not available, or there would be no need for a trial. It is precisely because pilot studies are so frequently wrong in indicating the superiority of new treatments, that RCTs need to be performed. Gilbert et al.[17] report a review of 46 randomised trials of innovations in surgery and anaesthesia, where only six of the new therapies studied were judged highly preferred compared with standard treatment (and in 22 studies, the standard treatment was found to be better). The harm done in the past, when treatments were accepted without proof of relative efficacy, can easily be demonstrated. Certainty about treatment recommendations is unusual in current medical practice, and cancer therapy provides a good example of this. In it, the level of uncertainty when dealing with an individual patient is extremely high. It is a relatively rare event that the chances of cure, and of complications from a form of treatment, are known precisely; an example is the point made by Botros[18] that prior to trial "researchers cannot give unbiased estimates for the survival rates of mastectomy as against lumpectomy". Moreover, it is always an impossibility to know exactly what the fate of the individual patient, facing these imperfectly known odds, will be. Are patients who accept randomised assignment to treatment in a carefully controlled trial being asked to accept higher risks of harm than those who choose between the same standard or experimental therapy outside of the study? The risk *inherent* to the treatment is not influenced by whether it is chosen or assigned; randomisation *per se* cannot alter these as yet uncompared risks. Refusal to accept random assignment to treatment leads to the same risks as the study patient faces; either the risk of not receiving an additional chance of cure or well-being (if standard treatment is chosen), or the risk of complications as yet unknown (if experimental therapy is elected). The randomisation is merely a device whereby the influence of different treatments on these risks can be determined and quantified.

It may also be considered unjust that the patient in a randomised trial does not have the ability to exercise choice in treatment options, where patients uninvolved in studies do. However, the information necessary for a really informed choice of treatment is not available to patients (or their doctors), else a trial need not be conducted. As Botros again asserts,[19] "The claim that there is frequently a best treatment for a patient, when taking into account quality of life, besides survival and recurrence . . . should not be confused with the claim that a doctor can already tell before an RCT which is that treatment." Patients who are made aware of this, and agree to participation in a trial, exercise just as much *real* choice regarding their treatment (given that the data required for an adequately informed choice are not available to patient or researcher alike) as those who select therapy outside a study.

Is patient autonomy respected when treatment is randomly assigned? It could be argued that the consent to becoming a subject in an RCT is in effect a waiver of the exercise of autonomous choice, a denial of one's own relevant attitudes and valuations of treatment. However, the patient who is fully informed about the research, its design, and its rationale, and who willingly agrees to participate, in making that choice to be enrolled exercises more autonomy than in choosing to accept or reject "standard" treatment by hunch or belief or personal preference (as no evidence of superiority of either therapy is established).

A related apparent difficulty which Botros discusses in her paper is the question of whether an autonomous patient, by giving informed consent to entry into a randomised controlled trial, can waive the right not to be used by others merely for their ends (and thus relieve the physician of the duty of beneficence). She concludes[20] that informed consent can only fulfil that function if a new, "choice conception of rights" model is applicable to the doctor-patient relationship. I would argue, however, that such a "choice conception of rights" model is in fact the one currently accepted; both legally and theoretically, the competent patient's decision to refuse that which is beneficial and recommended is respected—and autonomy *is* regarded as capable of overriding considerations of beneficence. The argument could be taken further, however, and her underlying premise questioned, i.e. that RCTs test medical procedures which are primarily aimed at benefiting future, not current, patients. It is true that in other forms of human experimentation, the subject has no or little chance of benefit; in Phase 2 trials of cancer therapy, for example, some benefit may result for the subject, but the aim is to improve the treatment of others in the future. In Phase 3 RCTs, though, the first, foremost, and overwhelming goal is the provision of the best possible health care to the patient, which remains the goal whether or not the patient chooses to participate in the study. The proposal of entry into a controlled study is an admission by the physician that the ideal of recommending the best known therapy cannot yet be achieved; being honest about the current state of medical knowledge is surely not an abrogation of the doctor's duty to the patient, but part of it. That being the case, the doctor's subsequent duty becomes the implementation of the plan for treatment which has been decided upon, and appropriate support during this treatment; and this duty remains the same whether treatment is taking place on or off study (although the careful monitoring and assessment of patients treated in an RCT tends to improve the quality of their treatment, not diminish it). Thus we cannot recognise that the purpose of obtaining informed consent to RCTs of therapy is to "absolve" the physician of the duty of best possible care; this duty still applies and is fulfilled within otherwise ethically acceptable Phase 3 trials. Consent to treatment in a randomised trial has the same role as consent to other treatment, namely assurance that coercion, deceit, or manipulation have not been used, and truthful information provided, in putting the patient in a position to make autonomous choices about therapy.

Another ethical problem in RCT design is the use of controls, which sometimes, where no effective therapy is known to exist, will consist of patients who are untreated, but who receive placebo "therapy". Issues of deception have been raised in the past, where patients were not informed that there was a possibility of assignment to placebo; but these concerns can be overcome if patients are made aware of the possibility that they may receive a pharmacologically inactive agent, and at the same time educated as to the reasons for this. Patients and physicians both are biased in favour of wishing all patients to receive some form of active therapy; and double-blind design, where neither the patient nor the physician knows which arm the patient has been assigned to, ensures that these biases toward active therapy do not impact on the patient's care and the doctor's enthusiasm. It is not just fidelity to research design that makes the use of placebo controls so important. It is because the reason for RCTs is to treat current patients in such a way that they are not harmed, and better recommendations to future patients will result. Only this, the ability to incorporate the knowledge gained into improved clinical policy, can justify the appeal to the altruism of the trial subjects. On a practical level, then, making sure that the results of clinical trials are actually accepted and used is as much an ethical obligation as their original design. Where neither clinicians nor researchers have been able to establish the relative merit of any form of therapy over none in the past, it is imperative to use such a "no-therapy" arm in current trials. By doing so, the patient is not deprived of anything known to be of value (including the doctor's supportive care and enthusiasm for the supposed treatment, be it active or placebo), where a double-blind design is used.

Problems relating to equipoise

Although a problem arising directly out of randomised controlled trial design, we should consider it separately as it represents, arguably, the thorniest of the dilemmas facing the doctors and patients involved.

The format in which RCTs are designed requires the proposal of a null hypothesis, i.e. that the two methods of treatment under consideration will lead to equal results with respect to the endpoint chosen—be it survival, response rates, recurrence rates, etc. One then tests this, during or at completion of the trial, and sees if the treatments have achieved equal results. When one arm of the trial shows apparently better results, one only accepts that this has disproved the null hypothesis, and that the difference in results is significant, when a convincingly low level of risk that the difference has occurred by chance can be demonstrated. A safe level of risk, that is commonly relied on in RCT design, is a probability of less than 0.05, in other words that there is a risk of only 1 in 20 that the apparent difference is due to chance.

The initiation of a trial thus requires that the participants begin by assuming no difference between the treatment arms. In order to think it right for patients to receive either of the two treatment options, the doctor must believe that neither treatment is superior. But of course, in order to think there is merit in organising such a study at all, there must be good reason to hope that one of the arms is likely to be better—either because of a greater success rate in cure or control of disease, or because it would result in a lower complication rate with the same chance of cure or control. What ethical significance does this "good reason to hope" have? Does it in fact prevent the clinician from really being able to assume no difference between the treatment options? Or does the knowledge that these hopes will frequently be false allow the doctor to ethically allow patients to receive the treatment he or she has reason to believe will not be as effective (though no valid proof exists one way or the other)?

That state of genuine uncertainty regarding the relative merits of two treatments under consideration is referred to as *equipoise* (from "the state of equal weights on a balance; a position of equilibrium"). The crucial ethical questions revolve around how we determine what genuine uncertainty must be, and whether the uncertainty of others should influence the investigator's position.

For example, if historical data, usual practice, hunch, or modality bias lead a physician to be "certain" that one form of management is superior, a restrictive definition of equipoise (demanding that the doctor can find *no* reason, scientifically valid or not, to choose between the therapies) would suggest that this physician could not ethically enrol patients in an RCT comparing that treatment which he prefers to another. An unacceptable corollary of this definition of equipoise, however, is that it entails widening of the scope of "standard" therapy felt to be ethically correct. We would be led to accepting that poorly informed, uncritical, biased doctors, offering treatment they believe is in their patients' best interests (despite the great harm which may result), are ethically equivalent to the well informed and honest physicians who might treat patients very differently, or who may have the honesty to see that their treatment preferences are not validly based, and thus propose trials to improve this situation. Given the unsatisfactory basis and provisional nature of most medical "knowledge", there is great intellectual dishonesty and hubris implied, when rejecting stringent scientific standards for treatment recommendations. A wider definition of equipoise is, therefore, more consistent with the doctor's duty to offer the best possible treatment to the patient—and Freedman's definition[21] of clinical equipoise is perhaps the appropriate one to employ when assessing the moral permissibility of offering patients random assignment to one of two treatments. He defines it as the state of affairs where there is no consensus within the expert clinical community about the comparative merits of the alternatives to be tested. Using this criterion, the ideal of medical practice outlined earlier in the introduction to this paper is likelier to be attained; the ethical obligation is no longer expressed as "offer the patient the best treatment in your opinion", but "offer the patient the treatment considered to be best by the expert community using valid tests of merit". Byrne[22] expresses this another way when commenting on the "position of reflectiveness" of modern medicine with respect to its sources of evidence. He comments on increasing professional awareness that "all judgements are fallible and many positively mistaken", and thus where a rational treatment preference cannot be supported prior to trial, a problem of nonmaleficence does not exist.

But should the absence of expert agreement absolve the individual clinician from the responsibility of deciding on the acceptability of certain treatments? For patients not being treated in an RCT, that responsibility continues unchanged; why should it be any less when the patient is in a random assignment protocol? My response is that the *level of responsibility* for treatment assessment does not change; but that when there are no reliable criteria for making that assessment, the best exercise of responsibility is to attempt to develop them, by treating patients in a way (i.e. in an RCT) that will eventually make this possible, while still acting in their best interests.

An even more difficult question of equipoise involves devising stopping rules for trials in progress. Generally, accrual takes place over months or years, and interim analysis of the results of treatment would seem to be ethically imperative, so that we avoid doing harm or failing to do good to those patients who would be randomised to the treatment arm now shown to be inferior. Applying this principle leads to a dilemma: at what point in a trend toward superiority of one treatment over another do we feel it is unethical to continue randomising patients to both? This problem is compounded by the frequent occurrence in cancer therapy trials of the reversal of early trends toward benefit; and both late relapses and delayed serious complications make firm conclusions from interim analysis dangerous. The competing ethical demand to prevent premature closure of trials thus has a twofold basis: to prevent unwarranted failure to adopt treatment that truly is of benefit, because the scientific community is not persuaded that adequate significance levels have been reached to recommend it; and to avoid the premature adoption as standard treatment of an intervention which final analysis will show to have been of no benefit or harmful. Both are likely outcomes (many examples can be found in the clinical oncology literature), and it will never be possible within a given trial to know which (if either) will prove to be the case. The least risky course of action, arguably, for both the current patients and the future patients who will become beneficiaries of the research, is to continue accrual until a pre-decided level of statistical difference is attained, or until the planned full numbers of patients have been reached. Given the vagaries of human sympathy and bias, this plan is much likelier to be adhered to if an independent monitoring committee, rather than the investigators themselves, are performing the analysis of trends.

But does not respect for the patients' autonomy mandate that prospective study candidates be told of current trends before deciding to participate? It does not (although this is a position which causes us some concern); the purpose of continuing a trial, in the face of a trend to benefit of one of the treatments, is in part to prevent harm *to those enrolling*, from their being misled, as well as to future patients. Respecting study patients' autonomy would also require informing them that neither they, nor their doctor, will be aware of interim analysis results, and the reasons why this should be the case. Thus, full honesty is maintained between clinician–researcher and patient–subject, at the cost of a small risk of harm. This is not a completely satisfactory solution, as the possibility remains that study patients are being asked to agree to an admittedly small (but not zero) chance of potentially avoidable harm, for the sake not only of their own protection, but also in the interests of the patients of tomorrow. This is not at the level of using patients as a mere means; but avoiding the risk of potentially preventable harm, no matter how small, remains an essential ethical task which perhaps is not always being adequately attempted here. This may, however, end up by being a compromise which patients and society are willing to make for the sake of the greater good for the community, even if only for the potential good of the individual involved. It may come to be considered on an ethical par with the risks patients face when being treated in teaching hospitals. The trainee's undeniable need to learn to take responsibility and perform procedures unsupervised remains a mixed blessing to the patient on the receiving end.

The regulation of randomised clinical trials of therapy

It will have become clear from the above ethical analysis of RCTs, that there are no features which are intrinsically incompatible with respect for the rights and interests of the patients who would take part. Research subjects do share in the expressed ends of these research efforts, and the inherent risks (with the possible exception of agreed non-disclosure of interim analyses) are no more, and generally much less, than those which are intrinsic to any medical intervention. The potential benefits to future patients, and all society, if such studies can be done without ethical compromise for the test patients, are enormous.

It is obvious, though, that when researchers become persuaded of the potential good of research, and where some career goals may be linked to performing it, the risks of corners being cut and safeguards of autonomy being neglected are real. The question of how best to regulate clinical investigations, in order to keep these risks at a minimum, and to ensure optimal standards of design and clinical usefulness, is a difficult one. The dangers of overregulation include the possibility that much needed research will not get done, as the bureaucratic red tape and time consuming applications will be a major deterrent. This could be true, even of valuable studies, with acceptable risks, to which patients would have had no difficulty in consenting. There is also the theoretical possibility that where excessive numbers of rules are in place, the individual researchers are led to abandoning their personal responsibility for ethical decision-making, as they may assume that compliance with the rules must always ensure that no ethical conflict is present.

The dangers of underregulation are probably more acute. The possibility that patients' rights will not be respected increases, and trials involving unacceptably high risks to patients may be allowed to proceed. With very little regulation, neither the public nor the health care profession may become sufficiently aware of the ethical dimensions to RCTs.

An attempt has been made in this paper to formulate the best compromise between these two poles. The minimal regulatory control should be exerted at the macro level (i.e. nationally or internationally). International and national codes must retain the flexibility and inclusiveness which allows them both to guide current research practice, and to stimulate debate as to its improvement. The more restrictive and rigid rules, which can lead to sanctions if flouted, are only appropriate at a micro level (i.e. hospital, research unit, or community). Such rules are only likely to apply to local problems if they arise out of a consensus search to deal with them; the use of ethical committees, with the ultimate power of sanction being the right to refuse permission for the proposed research, can be an effective approach. This, coupled with the meso level of regulation provided by the granting agencies' possible refusal of funds where ethical standards are not met, should provide adequate regulation of the ethics, and the scientific merit, of clinical trials. That the public, the health care professions, patients, lawyers, and philosophers have many opinions about the weighting of the ethical principles involved, leads me to recommend both a wide representation of opinion and background on ethical committees, and the enforced infusion of new blood into them at regular intervals. That their composition must include fair representation both from physicians and other health care workers, and from non-medical professionals, will ensure the benefits of self-regulation (familiarity with the issues, better understanding of all aspects of the risk/benefit ratios, the encouragement of personal responsibility for the research proposed), and of "other"-regulation (alternative viewpoints, less bias).

Further, the common law *ought* to provide the same legal support for informed consent provisions, and for negligence in treatment, both in the therapeutic research context, and in ordinary medical practice; the standards ought not to be different between the two. The likelihood of a court case to test the required standard of information for consent is very small, however; this makes the work of hospital ethical committees in encouraging fully informed consent all the more vital.

There is only one area where national legislation could play a useful role. This is in the establishment of a system of reparation for those who are harmed by unforeseen hazards of being in a research protocol. These victims have no possibility of success in a civil negligence suit as duty of care was not breached. A legislated no-fault research compensation fund would both give them recourse to source of just recompense for their altruism and suffering, and might also increase accrual to trials, if the worry that unpredictable serious complications cannot be compensated is keeping some otherwise willing volunteers out of clinical research now.

Conclusion

It is frequently argued that in examining the ethics of the randomised controlled trial, a conflict can be seen to exist between the needs of society and those of the individual patient. The traditional nature of the doctor–patient covenant, i.e. that the doctor pledges to offer the patient that treatment which the doctor thinks best, is felt to safeguard the principles of maximising benefit and avoiding harm, while offering the best chance of maintaining respect for the individual. If the doctor's opinion is based on scientifically validated knowledge and experience, we would agree that this covenant is ideal; but we should favour, instead, the paradigm for medical practice which requires that the doctor's own opinion be influenced by, or in some circumstances subservient to, the standard of proof required by the expert community. This model, after all, does mirror the way in which the uneducated opinions of the medical student (no less well meaning than the licensed practitioner) become, through exposure to the medical community, representative of its standards. What is really called for is the adoption by practitioners of an even higher standard of proof of validity in therapeutics than was required during their training.

This paper has set out to show that the risks are minimal in participating in an RCT which is scientifically sound, which asks a valid question, where there is no prior established knowledge of the relative merits of the treatments in question, and where preliminary results are independently monitored according to pre-agreed rules. There is no doubt that the goals of minimising harm and doing good are well served by treating patients within a trial framework, and there is much truth to Brewin's assertion that "a doctor who contributes to randomised treatment trials should not be thought of as a research worker, but simply as a clinician with an ethical duty to his patients not to go on giving them treatments without doing everything possible to assess their true worth".[23] The closer we come to being able to provide full information and free choice to potential research subjects, the more their dignity and individual worth is preserved.

The same ideals which motivate caring for the sick and attempting to cure disease are at work in our desire to achieve medical progress. There is no inherent battle between society's demand for this progress, and the rights of individual patients. Society is no nameless, faceless, amorphous "thing". It is individual persons, pure and simple, who are just as entitled to the respect for personhood, freedom from harm, hope for benefit, and progress toward justice as the current patient. If beneficence and respect are valid ethical principles in the relationship between individual doctor and patient, then they must be seen as just as valid for the individuals who make up society. If we see compelling reasons to try to ease the suffering and attempt the cure of present day patients, there are equally strong reasons to improve the lot of future patients. Physicians have a duty to recommend and provide the best possible therapy and can only fulfil this duty where validation of its worth is possible; this entails combining research and practice in a way which benefits both the current patient and those in the future. This is the mandate for the form of human experimentation this paper has been considering; it derives from the duty to the patient which has always been the cornerstone of medical ethics.

Notes and references

1. David J. Rothman, "Ethics and human experimentation—Henry Beecher revisited" (1987) 317 *New England Journal of Medicine* 1195-9.
2. Peter Armitage, "Controversies and achievements in clinical trials" (1984) 5 *Controlled Clinical Trials* 67-72.
3. Stuart J. Pocock, *Clinical Trials: A Practical Approach* (New York: J. Wiley and Sons, 1983).
4. William A. Silverman, "The ethics of human experimentation", in *Human Experimentation: A Guided Step into the Unknown* (Oxford: Oxford Medical Publications, 1985).
5. H. Tristram Engelhardt Jr, "Diagnosing well and treating prudently: randomized clinical trials and the problem of knowing truly", in S. F. Spicker *et al.* eds, *The Use of Human Beings in Research* (Dordrecht, Netherlands: Kluwer Academic Publishers, 1988).
6. Hans Jonas, "Philosophical reflections on experimenting with human subjects", in Paul A. Freund ed., *Experimentation with Human Subjects* (London: George Allen and Unwin, 1974).
7. Gustav Giertz, "Ethics of randomised clinical trials" (1980) 6 *Journal of Medical Ethics* 55-7.
8. Kathryn M. Taylor *et al.*, "Physicians' reasons for not entering eligible patients in a randomised clinical trial of surgery for breast cancer" (1984) 310 *New England Journal of Medicine* 1363-7.
9. Barrie R. Cassileth *et al.*, "Attitudes toward clinical trials among patients and the public" (1982) 248 *Journal of the American Medical Association* 969-70.
10. Nigel Kemp *et al.*, "Randomised clinical trials of cancer treatment—a public opinion survey" (1984) 10 *Clinical Oncology* 155-61.
11. Thurstan B. Brewin, "Consent to randomised treatment" (1982) 2 *Lancet* 919-21.
12. Nigel Kemp *et al.*, supra note 10.
13. Doris Penman *et al.*, "Informed consent for investigational chemotherapy: patients' and physicians' perceptions" (1984) 2 *Journal of Clinical Oncology* 849-55.
14. Arthur L. Caplan, "Is there an obligation to participate in biomedical research?", in S. F. Spicker *et al.*, eds, *The Use of Human Beings in Research* (Dordrecht, Netherlands: Kluwer Academic Publishers, 1988).
15. Barrie R. Cassileth *et al.*, "Informed consent—why are its goals

imperfectly realized?'' (1980) 302 *New England Journal of Medicine* 896–900.
16. Heather J. Sutherland *et al.,* ''Are we getting informed consent from patients with cancer?'' (1990) forthcoming (personal communication).
17. John P. Gilbert, ''Statistics and ethics in surgery and anesthesia'' (1977) 198 *Science* 684–9.
18. Sophie Botros, ''Equipoise, consent, and the ethics of randomised clinical trials'', in P. Byrne ed., *Ethics and Law in Health Care and Research* (Chichester: John Wiley and Sons, 1990).
19. Sophie Botros, ibid. at 13.
20. Ibid. at 20.
21. Benjamin Freedman, ''Equipoise and the ethics of clinical research'' (1987) 317 *New England Journal of Medicine* 141–5.
22. Peter Byrne, ''Medical research and the human subject', in Callagan and Dunstan eds, *Biomedical Ethics: an Anglo-American Dialogue* (New York Academy of Sciences, 1988).
23. Thurstan B. Brewin, supra note 11.

Legislative criteria: the Human Fertilisation and Embryology Bill *

John Habgood

The clauses concerning embryo research in the Human Fertilisation and Embryology Bill are controversial, and will go on being controversial, despite the large Parliamentary majorities in favour of allowing some research under strictly controlled conditions. Sharp disagreements of this kind usually reflect different ethical presuppositions. It may be useful, therefore, to set out in a very simple form the different types of question which provide the criteria for such decisions, and which may carry different weight in different ethical traditions. Broadly speaking, there are four types of question: those to do with *principles*, those to do with *consequences*, those to do with *precedents* and those to do with *motives*.

All are important in the attempt to find a broad ethical consensus on which to base legislation. To analyse a problem under these four headings does not necessarily make it any easier to agree. Discussions on contentious issues are rarely conclusive. But to understand why there are disagreements can take some of the sharpness out of debate, and help to remove misunderstandings. I intend to look at each area of questioning in turn, taking them in reverse order.

Editor's note: The Bill received the Royal Assent on 1 November 1990. Under the Human Fertilisation and Embryology Act, the Statutory Authority may grant licences for research on human embryos up to the 14th day of their development.

Motives

Good motives do not excuse actions which are wrong on other grounds. Equally, bad motives do not necessarily invalidate good actions, despite T. S. Eliot's strictures against doing "the right thing for the wrong reason". Personal motives may well have major moral significance in the assessment of individual actions, but in the realm of public policy, motives are frequently mixed and extremely difficult to assess. Where there is evidence to suspect bad motives, however, these can arouse justifiable suspicion about the ethical validity of a particular choice.

There are good motives for wanting to undertake embryo research, of which the most obvious is the desire to improve therapy and to enlarge the area of therapeutically useful knowledge. There are also good reasons for wanting to ban research, of which the most obvious is the desire to protect and value human life in all its forms, and at all stages of development. Researchers might claim that they too share this motive, though they work out its implications in a different way, just as the opponents of research would claim that they too are concerned with therapy, though not at the cost of what they see as human lives.

It is in the suspicions about bad motives that the discussion in this area of questioning becomes more acrimonious. Researchers, for instance, may suspect that opposition to their work is all part of an anti-science campaign, and fear that a total ban on research in a potentially fruitful field might deliver a body blow to scientific confidence. Anti-researchers retaliate by drawing parallels with Nazi experiments on human beings, and it is noteworthy that in the House of Lords debate on the second reading of the Bill, the most emotional speech, and the one which received the attention of the press, drew precisely this parallel. The thin end of the wedge argument is also widely canvassed, and it has been strongly argued that the 14 day limit for research will be quickly eroded, and that the researchers see this as a bridgehead rather than as a goal.

Accusations about hidden intentions have been most vociferous among the anti-researchers, and the following quotation from a leaflet published by the Society for the Protection of the Unborn Child is not untypical: "Using women's bodies as laboratories, and embryos as guinea pigs, will benefit principally the multi-national drug companies and the population controllers." It would be difficult to pack more loaded words into a single sentence, except perhaps in the final exhortation which decorated this particular leaflet: "Stop human vivisection now."

Recognition of honourable motives on both sides can help civilised debate. Unfortunately, though, honourable motives are not enough, nor is it possible to rely on them in practice as the sole safeguard against abuse, despite the fact that voluntary controls on embryo research in this country have hitherto worked reasonably well. A legislative framework is needed, and becomes all the more necessary, as research passes out of the hands of the pioneers into a more commercial context.

Precedents

Much decision-making begins with the questions, "What did we do last time?" and, "Are there any parallels?" In the field of embryo research there are no strong precedents. Abortion is perhaps the closest, because attitudes towards abortion expose beliefs about the moral status of the embryo and fetus. There is a long Christian tradition in which abortion has been condemned at any and every stage of development, but there has also been a recognition that its degree of seriousness as an offence increases as the fetus grows older. There has been, in other words, an implicit acknowledgement that the moral significance of the fetus is not identical at all stages, though there are some who would fiercely contest this point of view.

Although ethical thinking about abortion can give clues, therefore, as to how an embryo or a conceptus ought to be treated, the moral dilemma posed by research is significantly different. Abortion is essentially about a conflict of evils, and the choices are centred on a particular mother and child, either or both of whom stand to gain or lose. The dilemma posed by research concerns the use of a conceptus, which can only be destroyed in the process, for the future benefit of others. There is a conflict of evils, but it does not focus on particular individuals who face an immediate problem. The existence of such conflict cannot, therefore, be as easily used to justify an act of destruction in the case of research as in the case of abortion, and it is best therefore not to treat one as a precedent for the other.

There are more general precedents which might offer guidance, notably the history of the acceptance of many medical techniques which were once regarded as morally dubious. Transplant surgery, for instance, was once felt to violate the sense of human dignity and integrity just as, in an earlier generation, vaccination was condemned as entailing an "animalisation" of human beings. Similar feelings surfaced in the more recent proposal to use pigs' hearts in human transplants. On the whole, the experience has been that techniques once regarded as shocking cease to shock in a comparatively short space of time. This may be through a blunting of moral sensibilities. Equally, it may be a belated recognition that the shock was unnecessary, and that human dignity and integrity easily survive these apparent assaults.

However, the changes in feeling are not all in one direction. Greater sensitivities about animal experiments and growing worries about abortion may be the tip of a large iceberg. Many people are expressing fears about an increasingly reductionist view of human life. There are fears about opening the door to wider eugenic programmes. There are fears about commercial pressures once they gain a hold in what is a potentially lucrative field. Indeed, in the United States interest is already being expressed by some large companies in the possibilities of drug testing on spare embryos.

History shows that the boundaries of the acceptable are by no means fixed, and do not always move in a more liberal direction. The present Bill would limit some activities which are at present uncontrolled by law, and give legal recognition to others, for example the donation of gametes, which at present are not protected by law. It is as well to recognise slippery slopes in all directions.

The appeal to Christian tradition as a guide in these matters can draw on a strong and consistent desire to protect human life in all its forms, with a special emphasis on its weakest and most vulnerable forms. The element of uncertainty in the tradition, and the potential for disagreement, lies in the realm of definitions. Advances in embryology have provided some Christians with support for their claim that human life begins at an identifiable moment, namely fertilisation. This claim is put forward on the basis of Scripture and an unbroken historical tradition, despite the fact that human fertilisation was only described for the first time in 1875. Other Christians have questioned whether this story of human origins and this definition of human life is as clear as it seems, and stress instead the emergence of a single identifiable embryo as an episode in a complex story. I shall return to this disagreement later. The point I wish to make now is that there is no particular reason based explicitly in Christian tradition for deciding in favour of one side or the other.

Direct appeals to such Scriptural texts as Psalm 139 and Jeremiah 15, do not carry conviction, even if it were reasonable to suppose that the Scriptures are intended to give us detailed knowledge about the processes of human formation. The obvious meaning of such texts is that God has foreknowledge of us, and there is no time at which we fall outside His loving purposes. It is illegitimate to look in them for a definition of when this process begins. The appeal made by some Christians to the story of the Anunciation to Mary, and the Virginal conception of Jesus, are equally dubious grounds for beliefs about embryology. Christians who assert in faith that these things happened are fortunately not required to say precisely how or when they happened, whereas it is precisely the how and when questions which are relevant to the moral issues under discussion.

To dismiss these specific Christian contributions to the debate is not to deny that there are serious questions to be considered about God's intentions in calling things to be. Can, or should, all potentials for life be realised? Or is the universe of a kind in which some frustration of potentials is inevitable? Lurking behind these questions, framed as they are in theological terms, are huge biologically-inspired questions about the significance of the fecundity of biological processes, and the corresponding problems of waste and destruction. It may be that God's intentions can only be seen with hindsight in the fulfilled potentiality of His creatures, rather than in the enormous quantity of unfulfilment which undergirds them.

Consequences

The assessment of the likely consequences of actions and policies is the most commonly cited basis for decision-making in the public sphere. Stated thus crudely, however, it does not take us very far. Every action may have endless consequences, and those consequences themselves need to be ethically evaluated. Some distinction needs to be made between relevant and irrelevant consequences, and this too may entail ethical judgment. There are useful distinctions between immediate and long-term consequences, and individual and social consequences. On the whole, long-term consequences and social ones are harder to predict than immediate and individual ones, and therefore tend to weigh less heavily in the decision-making process. Medicine has a strong bias towards immediate and individual conse-quences. Doctors tend to focus their concern on the patient and the illness immediately in front of them. Research and preventative medicine take the long-term perspective, but still have a bias towards the needs of individuals. The way in which individuals are influenced by their social context, and the ways in which this can be adversely affected by short-term decisions, are often important factors in a religiously based ethic, but can seem too nebulous to those who have immediate decisions to make.

Within the embryo debate, attempts have been made to justify very limited forms of research on a conceptus or embryo which is itself likely to benefit directly from the research being done on it. In practice the opportunities afforded for this kind of research are so limited as to be valueless. Furthermore, it suffers from the grave moral objection that the risks entailed in it are risks to an actual mother and child, risks entailed at the leading edge of research, and which cannot be assessed for safety in the absence of the less direct kind of research provided for in the Bill.

The main difficulty in predicting the long-term social conse-quences of disallowing research on embryos is that nobody can tell what research might achieve until it has actually been done. Given the fact that in-vitro fertilisation at present has a low success rate, it seems fairly safe to assume that, in the absence of further research, this will not be greatly improved; there would thus be a serious question mark over the ethical propriety of continuing to use such an imperfect technique. It also seems reasonable to assume that to forbid research in a particular area for reasons which were not seen by the researchers themselves to have ethical validity might further widen the gulf between scientists and the rest of the community, at a time when scientists themselves are already feeling undervalued.

The main long-term social consequence of allowing research might be a devaluation of human life, a further step in the long process of treating human beings as objects. On the other hand, if the aims of research are clearly therapeutic, and if the procedures clearly result in the birth of healthy babies to couples who have long been wanting them, then it could be argued that the social consequences of such research might be to increase the valuation of human life, by virtue of the heroic measures undertaken to produce it.

Similarly, it can be argued on the one hand that genetic selection at the pre-implantation stage devalues the lives of the disabled. But it can also be claimed that such selection might provide enormous help and encouragement to those who know they are the carriers of genetic defects, by greatly increasing their chances of bearing a normal child.

These arguments are tenuous. Most of them depend upon the way in which perceptions change as practices change. Furthermore, the setting up of legislative safeguards can in itself have a major influence on public attitudes. Effective control mechanisms can, in this respect, be as significant as outright prohibition; it does not follow, therefore, that long-term social considerations about human devaluation require the latter. As regards the more immediate consequences of research, the onus is on the researchers to demonstrate that their work has major therapeutic possibilities, and on the legislators to demonstrate the exceptional nature of the permission given to work in such a sensitive area.

Principles

Despite the fact that most decisions in the public sphere rest on an assessment of likely consequences, however difficult this might prove to be, the appeal to principles can, and in some circumstances must, have decisive weight. In the field of secular ethics Kant, as it were, acts as a corrective to Mill. In the Christian context, the belief that there are moral absolutes outweighs any argument from expediency.

The question is, therefore, whether embryo research violates a principle of such importance that all other considerations are irrelevant. Does research break the principle of respect for human life in such a way as to settle the matter? Or are the uncertainties in the application of this principle to the human conceptus so great as to open up the argument to all the other considerations which have so far been adduced? In what sense, in other words, can the conceptus be said to deserve the respect and protection given to a human being?

There need be no dispute over the fact that such a conceptus is human in a descriptive sense. It needs to be noted, however, that the word "human" is used both descriptively and evaluatively, and the former need not always entail the latter. It is an open question as to when something described as "human" needs to carry the full moral connotations of the word.

It is also clear that a conceptus forms part of a continuous history in which fertilisation is a decisive, but not the only decisive, event. Much of the technical argument about embryo research has focused on the earliest period of development at which genetic identity is fixed, but the cellular identity of the developing organism is not. In the stage of undifferentiated growth following fertilisation, any one of the large number of cells in the conceptus may develop into the embryo and, in some cases, into more than one embryo. To say that fertilisation is the beginning of a human life, therefore, as if from that moment human identity were fixed, is to over-simplify a confused and complex process.

The argument that, despite the fluidity of personal identity at this earliest stage, it is nevertheless reasonable to recognise and respect the potential of the developing organism is frequently stated and has considerable strength. Yet there is something logically strange about giving high valuation to potential, when there is as yet no clearly definable entity which possesses that potential, and before the conditions, notably implantation, have begun to be fulfilled through which alone that potential can be realised.

From a biological perspective, the significance of genetic union is that it provides a new source of information and sets in motion a process through which a new being, and ultimately a new person, is formed. This process is not simply an unfolding of what is already there, but is an actual process of creation through interactions both inside and outside the developing organism. From this perspective it makes little sense to say that at one moment there is a human being, whereas a few moments previously there was not. Biological processes are in general not amenable to such sharp distinctions, and therefore fit uncomfortably into legal definitions. If it is asked from a legal point of view whether a conceptus is a thing or a person, the only sensible answer is neither. It is an organism on the way to becoming a person. Given the right conditions its personhood will develop with the development of certain attributes, and the most basic and rudimentary of these is cellular identity which becomes fixed at around the time of the formation of the primitive streak.

Arguments from principle based on the nature of the conceptus are thus not as clear and straightforward as reliance on them to provide moral absolutes might suggest. This uncertainty corresponds to ordinary moral perceptions as evidenced, for example, in attitudes towards miscarriages. A miscarriage may be seen as a tragic event, and I would not wish in any way to underplay the sense of loss which might be felt after even a very early miscarriage. It is noticeable, however, that the fruits of the miscarriage are not generally treated with the respect due to a human life. The need for some kind of funeral service for still-born babies is achieving wider and wider recognition, but miscarriages are usually flushed away down the drain without much sense that this is inappropriate or disrespectful. As in the case of abortion, there seems to be a sliding scale on which the intrinsic value of the growing fetus is acknowledged as the relationship between mother and unborn child develops, and there seems to be something curiously artificial about acknowledging full human value in a conceptus which has not even been implanted.

Should not its unique, genetic constitution, however, invite respect? Here again, it is important to distinguish between such a unique genetic constitution and personal identity. Identical twins have the same genetic constitution, but are different people. Genetic uniqueness is certainly significant in retrospect. Each of us is what we are by reason of a chance configuration of genes among billions and billions of possibilities. It does not follow, however, that every one of those possibilities has to be treated as potentially of infinite value before any unique attributes of an individual have actually begun to develop. Here, as earlier, arguments from potential seem to me to try to prove too much. Biological processes entail selection from among vast stores of potential, and it is only in the processes following this selection that distinctive value begins to emerge.

A zygote formed *in vitro*, and isolated for purposes of research outside the context of a personal life history and set of personal relationships, belongs within a context where only very limited potential will or can be fulfilled. Its intrinsic value is not that of a person, though neither is it negligible. Restrictive legislation concerning its treatment can help to strengthen our perceptions of it as belonging within the total mystery of human life, while not giving it so much moral significance as to override all other considerations about what may be done with it.

There is no certainty about moral decision-making in this complex area. We are right to be cautious. We are right also to remember that embryo research has been in progress for about twenty years without obvious abuse and, for the first time, we are imposing legal restrictions on it. I am not persuaded that the case against research is so strong as to require absolute prohibition, and although I believe that some of the moral argument in the Warnock Report side-stepped the major issues, the actual proposals in the Report in my judgment got the balance about right.

The legal status of the frozen human embryo

Andrew Grubb

Speaking in the House of Lords on 6 February 1990 Lord Hailsham of St Marylebone said:[1]

"An embryo is not a chattel . . . A human entity which is living is not a chattel and neither is it a person in any ordinary sense . . . It is wrong to try to define a human embryo in terms of established legal definitions which are plainly inapplicable to human embryos. Why must an embryo be one or the other? Why cannot it be just an embryo?"

The occasion for this comment was in response to an amendment moved in the House to the Human Fertilisation and Embryology Bill which sought to define the legal status of the embryo either as a person or a chattel according to their Lordships' preference. In the result the amendment was withdrawn.

What, then, is the legal status of a human embryo? Is it a person or is it property (a chattel) or does it have some, as yet, unarticulated legal status lying somewhere in between? Would, for example, someone wishing to bring a frozen embryo into the country need a passport or a customs declaration form? Could the frozen embryo of an immigrant enter the country as a dependent child of the immigrant or as hand luggage?

It is well known that in-vitro fertilisation (IVF) techniques have come to the aid of many infertile couples as a last hope for a child. The ability of doctors to extract and fertilise a human egg outside the body and return the resulting embryo to a woman who would be otherwise infertile has captured our imaginations. IVF techniques usually produce a surplus of embryos which are not immediately transferred to the woman who is undergoing the infertility treatment. It is common practice in IVF treatment to superovulate the patient and to fertilise any excess eggs. This has several advantages, amongst them that stored embryos may be used in subsequent treatments if treatment is initially unsuccessful without the need for the patient to undergo further laparoscopic egg retrievals. The excess embryos are stored in liquid nitrogen at very low temperatures. The success rate on thawing is far from perfect but it is now accepted practice to freeze the excess embryos. In addition to the embryos being used in subsequent treatment cycles, they could, if success is initially achieved, be used in the treatment of another infertile woman (embryo donation) or for research or simply be left to perish.

A number of situations may arise where the legal status of the embryo would be crucial in determining its fate. The most universal is probably the issue of research on human embryos. Much of the moral and legal debate has concentrated on this.[2] Can destructive research be justified? Status arguments are often prayed in aid by the protagonists in this debate. How can such research be permitted by the law if an embryo was a person? Embryo destruction would be murder. An unlikely position for the law to adopt but not one without its supporters.

But, in practical terms the legal status of the human embryo will arise in relation to the control and disposition of embryos, usually held in storage. Who has the power (or perhaps right) to decide on their fate and on what basis must any decision be made? A number of examples will help to set the scene. As we shall see subsequently, these are by no means the only difficult situations which could arise (see discussion of the Human Fertilisation and Embryology Act 1990 below).

1. A couple undergo infertility treatment and *disagree with the storage authority* about what should become of the excess stored embryos. For example, the couple wish to take their embryos somewhere else because the treatment they are receiving with their doctor at this centre proves unsuccessful (based on *York* v. *Jones* (1989) 717 F Supp 421).
2. A couple *disagree amongst themselves* on the fate of their

embryos. Their initial desire to receive treatment may, for one of the couple, cease to operate. The woman still wants to have a baby; the man does not. What should the fate of the stored embryos be? Whose decision should prevail?

3. The couple's disagreement may manifest itself in *divorce proceedings* and the courts may have to resolve a dispute over the embryos' fate in the context of a divorce case. Should the court treat the embryos as matrimonial property or matrimonial offspring? (based on *Davis* v. *Davis* (1989) 15 FLR 2097).

4. One or both of the couple *die*. Should the survivor have control over the stored embryos and what should happen if both die? Can an embryo be left to another in a will? Also, the possibility of posthumous implantation and birth raises the problem of inheritance, possibly long after the death of the gamete providers (based on the *Rios* orphan case in California/Australia).

If an embryo is a person in law and is entitled to the legal rights which flow from that, perhaps quite different resolutions of the above situations might present themselves than if the embryo were seen as a chattel or piece of property. Certainly it is commonly assumed that if an embryo is a chattel the dispositional authority will vest in the couple who provided the gametes and will be very wide indeed in scope. The couple could, for example, prima facie seek the return of their embryos from a storage body. They could determine in advance effectively the fate of their embryo even in circumstances of disagreement. And, of course, a survivor (if one died) would have sole dispositional authority and embryos could be bequeathed to another by will.

On the other hand, if the embryo is a person 'dispositional authority' would presumably again vest in the couple, but as with the power of parents over their children, the authority could only be exercised in the best interests of the embryo-person.[3] Care and control would now be a more appropriate and better description of the couple's powers over the embryo and there would be no question of an unlimited authority. Bequeathing an embryo to another by will would be unthinkable.

As one might expect English law has never had to consider the legal status of the extra-corporeal embryo. Lord Hailsham's statement set out at the beginning of this paper suggests that an embryo is an embryo; in other words it has a *sui generis* legal status. Clearly, he thought it was neither a person nor a chattel. He offered no reasons for this new third legal category of thing or object—no word exists to describe it. No such alternative category is known to law. When a court is seized of a case raising one of the situations the court would have no choice but to treat an extra-corporeal embryo as either *a person or a chattel*. The likely outcome would be that it would be held to be a chattel. Such law that exists points in this direction and the pragmatism of the common law would see that to treat an extra-corporeal embryo as a chattel is more consistent with common-sense than for it to be given the rights of a person.

Is an embryo a legal person?

The argument that an embryo is a legal person is based upon the proposition that life begins at conception when a genetically unique entity, with the potential for development into one of us, comes into existence. We are all familiar with this argument and with the sincerity of those who believe in it and advocate it as a doctrinal position for formulating law and public policy.

One court in the United States of America has adopted the proposition that life begins at conception[4] and the legislatures of Missouri and Louisiana have also statutorily adopted it.[5] Louisiana, for example, in 1986 conferred upon extra-corporeal embryos the status of a "juridical person" incapable of ownership.[6] The law also confers upon the embryo the right to be implanted and hence given a chance of development into a fetus and ultimately a baby.[7] In *Davis* v. *Davis*[8] seven embryos were held in storage. The couple, Junior and Mary Sue Davis, had undergone IVF treatment without success. The couple decided to divorce and the court was called upon to determine the fate of the seven frozen embryos. Mary Sue wished to obtain control of them so that they could be introduced into her with the hope of her becoming pregnant. Junior Davis, on the other hand, resisted her attempt because he did not wish to become a father. The trial court in Tennessee awarded temporary custody of the embryos to Mary Sue on the basis that they were in law persons because life began at conception. The court determined that the embryos' best interests lay in life and not death and so, as the judge put it,[9] "the manifest best interest of the children, in vitro, [is] that they be made available for implantation to assure their opportunity for live birth; implantation is their sole and only hope for survival".

The biological reality added to the philosophical imperative gave rise to a legal determination that embryos were persons. Once this was decided, the judge's ruling was inevitable. Life is almost always better than death or non-existence and since, in effect, Junior Davis was in favour of non-existence and Mary Sue wanted life for the embryos it was she who had to win.

We could say that *Davis* v. *Davis* is one of those American cases where, as Lord Hailsham put it in the debate in the House of Lords, "they ask[ed] themselves a silly question and then gave a foolish answer."[10] No doubt this would be his view of *Davis* v. *Davis*. But, on reflection, there is no silliness in the question "what should be the fate of the frozen embryos?" Nor necessarily is there any foolishness in the answer that their custody should be awarded to Mary Sue Davis. Instead, the defect in the judgment lies in the reasoning process which equates biological life with legal personhood and, as a consequence, treats embryos and children alike. That transition is a *non sequitur*. The case could have been decided the same way if the judge had adopted a property or chattel analysis. Such an analysis would vest decisional control in the procreating couple (subject to limitations on grounds of public policy). In the absence of a controlling statement about what should happen to the embryos in the case of disagreement or divorce, the court must make a decision based upon the relative equities of the parties.[11] In particular, the burden of unwanted fatherhood against the burdens of future alternative procedures for achieving pregnancy. There was no prior agreement in this case and the judge could have decided that the financial and emotional burdens of unwanted fatherhood for Junior Davis were outweighed by the burdens which would be placed upon Mary Sue if she had to undergo further egg retrieval and IVF procedures.

Subsequently, the Tennessee Court of Appeal overturned the trial judge's ruling and reached the rather curious result of granting both parties *joint* custody of the embryos.[12] The court refused to vest sole custody in Mary Sue Davis on the ground that Junior Davis had a constitutional right not to procreate. This would be infringed if his ex-wife was allowed to have their children against his wishes. The curiosity lies in the fact that their disagreement led to the court case in the first place and so joint custody solved nothing. The curiosity, however, disappears when it is noticed that, as the court pointed out in a footnote, Mary Sue had remarried and no longer wished to have the embryos implanted but was content that they should be donated to another infertile couple. Probably the Davis' could agree on this much.

Just because the factual problem evaporated in the *Davis* case does not mean that the reasoning of the trial judge could not be followed in a subsequent case. The "person analysis" adopted by him must lead a court to make a finding in favour of the party seeking to obtain the embryos for implantation whether it be the mother or the father. There is no room for flexibility and there is no room for manoeuvre. Added to which the knock-on consequences of the trial judge's reasoning make his position very unattractive for the normal pragmatism of the common law judge. Some of these consequences would be as follows:

— embryo research leading to death could be murder;
— embryos could not be harmed in any way; hence research of all kinds (except the purely observational) would be unlawful;
— inheritance rights would seem to exist even *before* implantation.

Whatever the merits of the medical/philosophical proposition that life/personhood begins at conception, apart from the *Davis* case the common law does not adopt it. A number of illustrations from different areas of English law establish this point.

Several decisions of the English courts have held that an unborn child is not a person in law. In two cases, *Paton* v. *BPAS*[13] and *C* v. *S*,[14] fathers sought injunctions to prevent their wife and girlfriend respectively from obtaining an abortion. In both cases they did not succeed.[15] One of the arguments presented in each case was that the unborn child was a legal person with capacity to sue and seek an injunction to prevent the proposed abortions. In both cases the courts held that an unborn child has no legal rights until it is born. In the *Paton* case Sir George Baker, the President of the Family Division, said[16]

"A foetus cannot, in English law, in my view, have any right of its own at least until it is born and has a separate existence from the mother. That permeates the whole of the civil law of this country . . ."

In *C* v. *S* Heilbron J approved this view[17] and noted that in certain circumstances prenatal injuries (i.e. those caused whilst in the womb) may be the subject of legal action by a child once it is born.[18] She observed that[19]

". . . the claim crystallises on the birth, at which date, but not before, the child attains the status of a legal persona, and thereupon can then exercise that legal right."

Similarly, in *Re F (in utero)*,[20] the Court of Appeal held that an unborn child lacked legal personality to be made a ward of court.

Each of these cases arguably involved a conflict between the interests (I deliberately do not use the word—rights) of the unborn child and the mother. But, in my view, it would be quite wrong to see the cases as only failing to recognise the legal status of the unborn child because to do so would lead to a certain conflict with the pregnant mother's interests. The decisions were not given on this narrower basis. If an unborn child is not a legal person, it cannot seriously be argued that a frozen two-, four- or eight-cell embryo is a legal person with all the legal consequences stemming from such recognition by the law.

A broad sweep of legal opinion throughout the world produces identical conclusions to those above. The Supreme Court of Canada,[21] the Supreme Court of the United States[22] and the High Court of Australia[23] have all decided that an unborn child (and hence I would argue a frozen embryo) is not a person in law.

Does the law of abortion provide any pointers as to the status of a fetus and hence, possibly, the embryo? What guidance we can obtain is, at best, inconclusive. Not surprisingly, the law of abortion has developed in an uneven way as politicians react to pragmatic considerations. It is correct to say that English law does provide some protection to unborn children through the legislation since abortion is a criminal offence unless a defence exists under the Abortion Act 1967.[24] The protection is not, however, universal nor uniform. If the fetus is less than 24 weeks gestational age, while the Abortion Act provides both procedural and substantive limitations on the availability of abortions,[25] abortions are still freely available.[26] Until 1991, a more mature fetus could not be aborted unless it was necessary to save the life of the mother.[27] In other words, considerable protection was given to a mature fetus.[28] However, the amendment to the Abortion Act by section 37 of the Human Fertilisation and Embryology Act 1990 permits an abortion even after 24 weeks on the so-called "fetal handicap" ground[29] or because of the danger of grave permanent injury to the mother's health[30] or risk to her life.[31].

Any protection that existed has been diluted by the 1990 amendments. Clearly, no rights are created here and even if there were, the fetus could not enforce them. Instead, what protections there are illustrate that the unborn child (with its potentiality for development into a live human being) is entitled to *some* protection against destructive acts and to an extent that protection increases with increasing maturity.[32] Ultimately however, little, if anything, can be gained from an analysis of the law of abortion to help in the search for the legal status of the embryo.

Is a frozen embryo property?

Defining an embryo as a legal person proves too much. It produces inconsistencies with the legal status of (and respect owed to) more developed forms of human conceptus. A property analysis may allow more flexibility and properly serve the needs of public policy in this area. On the other hand there are a number of strands of authority and arguments which point generally (and sometimes specifically) in the direction that frozen embryos are property and hence subject to the control of the procreating couple.

First, few would argue that human gametes—sperm and ova— were not susceptible to control through the gamete providers' rights in them as property.[33] The 1984 French case of Alain and Corinne Parpalaix illustrates this.[34] A French court ordered a sperm bank to return to Corinne Parpalaix the sperm of her dead husband which had been stored prior to his undergoing radiotherapy for testicular cancer which, subsequently, killed him.[35] In so doing, the court enforced an agreement between the storage authority and Alain Parpalaix "to preserve the sperm and restore it to the donor or to hand it over to the person for whom it was intended", i.e. his widow. Such a result is only consistent with the view that the sperm was property. In England, a slightly different analysis would be required. Of course, the Parpalaix case concerns a disposition upon death and, arguably, the sperm, as property, should pass to the surviving spouse under the rules of intestacy or, if a will existed, as part of the residuary bequest under the will. Strictly speaking, the agreement with the storage authority would only be a valid, enforceable, agreement *at the time of death* if it complied with the terms of the Wills Act 1837, i.e. it is properly witnessed etc.— which is unlikely.

Secondly, damage to or loss of sperm could give rise to an action in the tort of negligence for damage to or loss of property.[36] A donor who can prove that sperm or ova have been negligently damaged would have a legal claim, although the damages which a court would award might not be great unless the donor could establish that the loss was irreplaceable because, for example, he or she was now infertile.

Can it be different for embryos? Surely the genetic unification of the gametes to produce a unique human structure should not change our analysis completely? In a Federal Court case in New York in 1978 called *Del Zio* v. *Presbyterian Hospital*[37] the plaintiffs, a married couple, claimed damages for severe emotional distress and conversion (a property claim) after a doctor deliberately destroyed an embryo created from the couple's gametes in an IVF programme. Although the judge left both of the plaintiffs' claims to the jury, the jury only awarded damages on the emotional distress claim and not the conversion claim. In the result, therefore, the case is rather inconclusive on the issue of whether the embryo was viewed as property. Clearly, the judge thought so, otherwise he should not have left the issue to the jury but why they failed to award damages must remain a mystery.

Far clearer a judicial view can be seen in another Federal Court case decided in 1989, this time in Virginia called *York* v. *Jones.*[38] The Yorks underwent IVF treatment at a clinic in Virginia as a result of which one embryo was frozen and stored. After a number of unsuccessful procedures, the Yorks moved to California and asked the clinic to release the frozen embryo to them so that they could take it to a clinic in California. The Virginia clinic refused. The Yorks sued, claiming, amongst other things, a breach of contract and detinue (again a property based claim). The clinic sought to strike the Yorks' claim out as untenable but the judge refused. The judge held that in relation to both the contract and detinue claim the parties had created a bailment of the embryo by the Yorks to the clinic. Once the purpose of the bailment terminated, as it had when the Yorks did not seek any further treatment, the Yorks' proprietary rights to control the embryo entitled them to possession. The judge's language is an explicit recognition of the procreating couple's proprietary interests in a frozen embryo.

The decision is very significant indeed. It also illustrates something we shall return to shortly, namely the relevance of a couple's agreement as to the disposition of frozen embryos. In *York* v. *Jones* the terms of the agreement were considered by the judge as very important in recognising the proprietary rights of the couple in the embryo and, further, the scope of their continued authority in relation to its disposition once the agreement had been entered into.

If we pause for a moment, how would our reasoning differ if the French case had concerned frozen embryos? A surviving widow or widower would be entitled to exercise those rights over the embryo which the deceased partner could have exercised before his or her death as against the storage authority.[39] Dispositional control as against third parties must, as a matter of common-sense, vest in the gamete providers jointly or the survivor (or the survivor's estate if they die too). The right of control would, as a consequence, pass to the survivor.

Why not accept the property analysis?

However attractive it may sound, there is a general reluctance to accept the property analysis. A cluster of arguments are made. First, it seems inappropriate to vest ownership of a human embryo in anyone. Its *living* status together with its potential for development speak against a right of ownership. Secondly, there is the related argument that a property approach which entails ownership necessarily means that the couple have unlimited rights to control and dispose of human embryos, which is thought undesirable. For example, the Warnock Committee recommended that legislation should be enacted which would prevent ownership in a human embryo because that would be "undesirable".[40]

On reflection, these objections to the property analysis do not stand up to scrutiny. As to the first, it smacks of the philosophical argument that life begins at conception. In so far as the first objection is not based on this, it seems to object to the notion of ownership on some symbolic ground because of the inherent nature of living human material. While symbolism should not be undervalued—it may explain our reactions to cannibalism and corpse desecration—here it seems not to be sufficiently justified to elevate the human embryo out of the category of property and into the only other category known to law—that of a person. After all, ownership is only legal jargon for the ultimate source of the power of dominion and control over something else. Warnock, and indeed virtually every other body that has considered this issue, would give the couple, as the Report itself says, "rights to the use and disposal of the embryo, although these rights ought to be subject to limitation."[41] No other practical alternative can reasonably be suggested and sustained.

If we turn to the second objection and realise that it too is flawed, then the need to deny the property status of the embryo and its amenability to ownership (or at least control) is overcome. To accept that a frozen embryo is property does not entail the conclusion that the procreating couple can do what they like with the embryo. There will be limitations imposed on grounds of public policy. A court could take the view that the sale of an embryo was contrary to public policy and refuse to enforce a contract even though the Human Organs Transplant Act 1989 (which prohibits the sale of "organs") does not cover embryos.[42] Similarly, a court might consider the capricious destruction for no good reason or offensive disposal of an embryo to be contrary to public policy and refuse to enforce (or perhaps even enjoin) such conduct.

Take an example. A dog is property and I have control (derived here from ownership) over the animal and yet I may not treat it cruelly and I may destroy it but only humanely. We speak of having a sick animal "put down". Of course, these limitations on my rights are statutory in origin but that should not matter, they are merely manifestations of public policy limitations.

In the absence of legislative guidance, a court would, in my view, be entitled to decide that a couple's proprietary rights over a frozen embryo do not extend to destruction for no good reason. This would permit scientifically *justifiable* research on embryos of all kinds. Similarly, that destruction must be humane and compassionate. These latter two terms do not concede the argument that an embryo is a person because we readily use them in relation to animals, such as in the canine example. Permitting an embryo to thaw out and perish is different from flushing it down the laboratory sink or macerating it into tiny pieces. Of course these sorts of decision should properly be made by the legislature (and we shall see that some have already been dealt with in the 1990 Act), but the point is that the property analysis is not the evil (or "ugly sister" as Lord Hailsham called it[43]) that some would suggest. Orthodox legal analysis can take account of the special qualities that a human embryo possesses. The pragmatism of the common law could resolve the difficult situations of dispositional control of frozen embryos.

Applying the property analysis

A property analysis leads to the following general conclusion that dispositional control of a frozen embryo lies jointly with the couple whose gametes contribute to the embryo. If we recall the four situations mentioned earlier we can try and determine how a court would deal with each.

1. Donors versus storage authority

The first, you will recall, was exemplified by the case of *York* v. *Jones* in the US where a dispute arose between the couple and the storage body. In the absence of any prior agreement, the purpose underlying the bailment relationship created by the handing over of the embryos will cease to exist if the couple, for example, wish to take their embryos elsewhere. As with the American court, it is likely that an order for their return could be obtained. However, this simple case will rarely exist because of the existence of an agreement which may define some or all of the terms of the bailment relationship. In this context the embryo storage agreement will be all important.

Precisely what the status of any agreement would be will depend upon the circumstances. It could be contractual (outside National Health Service) or it could simply be an indication of the bailors' (the couple's) intentions. Would such agreements be binding even if contractual? Arguably, they would be binding providing two matters were satisfied: first, the terms of the agreement were sufficiently certain, and secondly, the couple and the storage body have acted to their detriment on the undertaking to create embryos on certain conditions.[44] The Interim Licensing Authority which "regulated" the use of modern reproductive techniques in infertility treatment between 1985 and 1991 recommended a specimen agreement which authorised the freezing and storage of excess embryos for up to two years, thereafter giving the storage body discretion to dispose of the frozen embryos by donation to another woman undergoing IVF treatment or by destroying them by approved methods.[45] Other than requiring 28 days' notice, the specimen agreement did not prevent the couple exercising their proprietary rights to regain possession during the two year period.[46] It seems likely, therefore, that an English court in such circumstances would reach the same conclusion as in *York* v. *Jones*. But necessarily, each decision must depend upon the specific agreement between the couple and the storage body.

2. Donor versus donor

If, however, the parties disagree with each other—the second situation identified earlier—the specimen agreement provides no answer. A court could simply split the property half and half between the parties but this would really suit no-one, particularly the party seeking to avoid parenthood. Instead, as we saw when considering the *Davis* case, the court should seek to make an equitable decision based upon the relative burdens of the parties in unwanted parenthood versus the burdens of further attempts to become pregnant under IVF procedures. In cases where the person seeking possession for implantation could undergo further egg retrieval or, if the male partner could find another procreating partner, arguably the burdens of unwanted parenthood are significant enough to outweigh the interests of the person seeking possession.[47]

3. Donor versus donor on divorce

The third situation—the *Davis* case itself—where the parties disagree and divorce, should be resolved in precisely the same way on the basis of this equitable distribution. Here, of course, any agreement would have no legal validity. A court would in a divorce case have no obligation to give effect to it.

4. On the death of one donor

The fourth situation, where one or both gamete providers die, can also be resolved on a property analysis satisfactorily. A survivor takes as of right as the survivor of joint property and could, of course, seek posthumous implantation although that would require the cooperation of a medical practitioner. If both die then the law of inheritance, whether testate or intestate, would apply. Unless specific provision is made in the law as Warnock recommended,[48] any subsequent implantation and birth of a posthumous embryo would, subject to adequate proof of parentage, give rise to a claim on the dead couple's estate.

The pragmatism and common-sense approach of the common law is more effectively furthered by a property analysis than one based upon the argument that an embryo is a person.

The Human Fertilisation and Embryology Act 1990

However, the discussion cannot end there because of the Human Fertilisation and Embryology Act 1990 (HUFEA) which received the Royal Assent on 1 November 1990. The Act creates a framework for the regulation of developments in embryology. Principally, this is achieved through the creation of the Human Fertilisation and Embryology Authority (the Authority). The Authority licenses infertility centres, research projects and storage facilities. The Authority replaced the Interim Licensing Authority (ILA), the self-regulating body created by the Medical Research Council and the Royal College of Obstetricians and Gynaecologists in 1985. Unlike the ILA, the Authority has statutory "teeth" to enforce the provisions of the Act and to enable it to carry out its licensing, monitoring and policing functions.

General scheme of schedule 3 of HUFEA

HUFEA does not explicitly spell out the legal status of the frozen embryo. Most of the relevant provisions of the proposed legislation are to be found in schedule 3, which creates a complex scheme whereby the consents of gamete providers determine the proper disposition, and define the power to control the use of human embryos. Paragraph 6(3) of schedule 3 of HUFEA prohibits the use for infertility treatment or for research of human embryos[49] created *in vitro* without the "effective consent" of both of the gamete providers.[50] Similarly, paragraph 8(2) provides that an embryo[51] created *in vitro* must not be kept in storage without the gamete providers' "effective consent".[52]

"Effective consent"

What is an "effective consent"? Paragraph 1 of schedule 3 defines it as a consent given in writing which has not been withdrawn by written notice[53] given to the person keeping the embryo (paragraph 4(1)).

When must an "effective consent" be obtained from the gamete providers? Prior to the creation *in vitro* of a human embryo, their consents must be obtained [54] as to its future use: (1) for infertility treatment of the gamete providers, (2) for infertility treatment of others, or (3) for research.[55] Further, if it is intended to store an embryo the gamete providers' consents must be obtained for this also.[56]

The consents to use or storage may specify conditions for the use of the embryos.[57] In addition, the gamete providers' consents to storage *must* specify what is to happen in *three* situations:

— what is to be the maximum period of storage if less than the statutory storage period which is five years for embryos;[58]
— what is to happen on the death of one of the gamete providers;
— what is to happen if one of the gamete providers should become mentally incompetent and unable to make decisions about the disposition of the embryos.

The provisions of schedule 3 vest dispositional control of human embryos[59] in the gamete providers jointly. Each has, in effect, a veto on the disposition (whether as to use or storage) of the product of his or her gametes. The provisions seek to determine the fate of an embryo from the date of its creation (subject to revocation or variation by the gamete providers).

What is the effect of HUFEA and when, if ever, does it not resolve an issue of control?

1. Agreement between the gamete providers

First, if the gamete providers continue to agree on the fate of the embryos their initial consents will determine what should happen to the embryos. However, this is subject to one situation: if the embryos remain in storage at the end of the statutory maximum storage period of five years, then the embryos must be "allowed to perish" (section 14(1)(c)). Here, we see legislative approval of the public policy restraints that might be placed upon dispositional control by requiring a humane and compassionate end to their existence.

2. Disagreement between the gamete providers

If the couple disagree and one or both withdraws their consent, then any use or continued storage (or any use or storage inconsistent with the varied consent) will not be in accordance with the statutorily required "effective consent" of both and so that use is prohibited or the storage must cease. The Act curiously does not specify in the case of a withdrawal of consent to storage what should then happen to the embryos. They cannot be kept until the storage period ends because of the explicit terms of paragraph 8(2) of schedule 3. Similarly, they cannot be returned to either spouse as part of fertility treatment unless they both agree. In any event, section 14(2) (b) prevents any supply of an embryo to another (including the gamete providers) once it has been stored except in the course of treatment services or to another licensed storage facility. The only option, therefore, is that the embryos must be allowed to perish. Indeed, this was the Lord Chancellor's view expressed during the course of the House of Lords' debate on the Bill.

3. Death of one or both of the gamete providers

If one or both of the procreating couple die, then continued storage (up to the statutory maximum) or disposal will follow as requested. It will be recalled that the fate of embryos in this situation is one of the *required* matters that must be dealt with by the gamete providers at the outset under paragraph 2(*b*) of schedule 3. The *Rios* orphan case in Australia in 1984[60] where both providers were killed in an aeroplane crash would be resolved under the Act by reference to the wishes of providers expressed in their initial consents. Unlike the legislative response in Victoria in Australia (where the case arose) that the Minister should direct their use in the infertility treatment of others,[61] the gamete providers' wishes will be determinative. If a surviving spouse then withdrew his or her consent to the specified use (or continued storage), the wishes of the deceased spouse would be overridden because, of course, *each* gamete provider has a veto on any use or storage.

What if one spouse attempted to leave an embryo to another in a will, for example, to a mistress? Could this raise the status of the embryo by requiring a court to determine whether it was property capable of being the subject of a testamentary disposition? Almost certainly it would not. A court would treat the 1990 Act as determining the fate of embryos on the death of one or both gamete providers. Hence, any purported disposition of an embryo as property in a will would not arise.

4. The gamete providers divorce: the Davis situation

What would happen if a *Davis* type case were to arise in England? If one of the gamete providers revoked his or her consent to the use or storage of the embryos, then an application of schedule 3 would appear to require the same course to be followed as in any other case where revocation of consent has occurred, i.e. situation 2 above. However, the solution may not be so simple. HUFEA does not purport to limit a divorce court's powers to reallocate matrimonial property or make orders concerning the custody of children of the marriage. It could be argued that the court would, as a consequence, have to decide whether a frozen embryo was matrimonial property or matrimonial offspring and make a decision concerning disposition on the basis of this determination.

On the other hand, the court could decide that the detailed provisions of HUFEA were intended to cover even the case of divorce. This is particularly likely if the Authority specifies, as it has power to do under paragraph 2(3) of schedule 3, that the gamete providers should in their consents specify what is to happen on their divorce. It is unlikely that an English court would embark upon the course of deciding whether an embryo was a chattel or a person unless it was unavoidable. Here, HUFEA provides an alternative ready-made solution. Disposition would be resolved applying the principles in situation 2 above.

5. Gamete providers disagree with storage body

The Act provides no enforcement provisions. How would a couple in the position of the Yorks fare in England if they sought the return of their frozen embryos from a storage body? If one (or both) revoked their consent to storage, under the Act, as we have seen, the embryos could no longer be held in storage. But, that does not mean they must be returned to the couple who provided the gametes. The Act is unhelpful because it does not explicitly provide for this contingency. A number of arguments need to be considered. Perhaps the gamete providers, if they were shrewd enough, could have dealt with this contingency by making it a condition of storage that they could seek the return of the embryos on giving reasonable notice. However, paragraph 8(2) probably only allows conditions relating to storage, not about the fate of the embryos when storage ceases. Equally, the embryos could not be used by others for any purpose because that can only be done in accordance with the consents of the gamete providers.

Hence, there are only two alternatives: either the embryos would have to be allowed to perish or they should be returned to the couple. If the storage body refused to return them could a court order be sought to obtain possession? The answer is that a court probably could not do this. Whatever the arguments about whether an embryo is a chattel or a person, section 14(1)(c) would prevent any claim for the return of the embryos because the couple would not be supplied with the embryo "in the course of providing treatment services" as is required by section 14(1)(c). There remains the possibility of transfer to another licensed facility if the gamete providers requested it. But, the Act does not impose a duty on the storage body to comply. Arguably, the storage body could refuse and the embryos would have to be "allowed to perish".

Conclusion

No statutory definition of the embryo's status was forthcoming from Parliament in HUFEA. Perhaps, it is unrealistic to expect Parliament to subject itself to facing up to more moral dilemmas in the near future. So, any suggestion that the Act should be amended to provide a definition is probably whistling in the wind. Arguably, as we have seen there is no need; the 1990 Act provides all the answers or, at least, can be interpreted by a court as doing so. However, the ingenuity of litigants and lawyers is always likely to provide further unspecified situations where status questions cannot be avoided by a court interpreting the Act as pre-empting the question of status. For example, could a tort action for destruction or loss of property be brought if an embryo was destroyed or damaged in storage or in a laboratory? A simple provision such as follows would achieve the desired goal:

"Subject to the provisions of this Act [HUFEA], in any court proceedings an extra-corporeal human embryo (whether frozen or otherwise) shall in law not be treated as a legal person but, instead, the court shall consider the embryo to be an entity amenable to the laws relating to personal property in so far as public policy does not otherwise require."

Until then, HUFEA provides many (perhaps all) of the answers but the question still has to be asked "What is the legal status of a frozen human embryo?" Is it a chattel or a person, or is it just an embryo?

Notes and references

1. (1990) 515 HL Deb Cols 750–1.
2. Botros, "Abortion, embryo research and foetal transplantation: their moral relationships" in P. Byrne ed., *Medicine, Ethics and the Value of Life* (Chichester: John Wiley, 1990). The literature is voluminous but some of it and the arguments are canvassed in Kennedy and Grubb, *Medical Law: Text and Materials* (Butterworths, 1989) chapter 8.
3. See the authoritative statements in the House of Lords in *Gillick* v. *West Norfolk and Wisbech AHA* [1985] 3 All ER 402. See now Children Act 1989, section 1 (the court).
4. *Davis* v. *Davis* (1989) 15 FLR 2097 (Tenn Cir Ct); on appeal [1990] WL 130807 (Tenn CA).
5. Missouri RS ss 1.205(1) (1986); Louisiana RS 9:ss 121–33. Some of the US legislation is discussed by Vetri, "Reproductive technologies and United States Law" (1988) 37 *International and Comparative Law Quarterly* 505.

6. Ibid., ss. 124 and 126.
7. Ibid. s. 130.
8. (1989) 15 FLR 2097 (Tenn Cir Ct) and [1990] WL 130807 (Ten CA, September 13, 1990).
   See the discussion in Robertson, "In the beginning: the legal status of early embryos" (1990) 76 *Virginia Law Review* 437.
9. Ibid.
10. Supra note 1.
11. See Robertson op. cit. note 8 at 473–83.
12. [1990] WL 130807 (Tenn CA, September 13, 1990).
13. [1979] 1 QB 276 (Baker P). Discussed in Kennedy, *Treat Me Right* (London: OUP, 1989) chapter 4.
14. [1988] 1 QB 135 (CA). Discussed in Grubb and Pearl, "Protecting the life of the unborn child" (1987) 103 *Law Quarterly Review* 340.
15. For a similar case in Canada see *Tremblay* v. *Daigle* (1990) 62 DLR (4th) 634 (Sup Ct).
16. Supra at 279.
17. Supra at 140.
18. Since July 1976 the action is created by section 1 of the Congenital Disabilities (Civil Liability) Act 1976. An action almost certainly could have been brought prior to this under the common law: *B* v. *Islington HA* [1991] 1 All ER 825 and *De Martell* v. *Merton & Sutton HA* [1991] 2 *Med LR* 209.
19. Supra at 140.
20. [1988] 2 All ER 193 (CA). Discussed in Grubb and Pearl, "Warding an unborn child" [1988] *Cambridge Law Journal* 362.
21. *Daigle* v. *Tremblay* (1990) 62 DLR (4th) 634. Notice also *Borowski* v. *Attorney General of Canada* [1987] 4 WWR 385 (Sask CA); on appeal to Supreme Court: (1989) 57 DLR (4th) 231 (dismissing appeal on procedural grounds).
22. *Roe* v. *Wade* 410 US 113 (1973).
23. *Attorney General (Qld) (ex rel Kerr)* v. *T* (1983) 46 ALR 275.
24. For a discussion of the legislation and its origins see Grubb, "Abortion Law in England—The Medicalization of a Crime" (1990) 18 *Law, Medicine and Health Care* 146.
25. For these see Grubb, ibid. The substantive limitations may not in reality exist, see Grubb, ibid. at 153–156.
26. See Grubb, "Abortion law—An English perspective" (1990) 20 *New Mexico Law Review* 649 at 658–668.
27. Infant Life (Preservation) Act 1929, section 1(1).
28. The Protection extended to a fetus "capable of being born alive" (section 1(1) of the Infant Life (Preservation) Act 1929). This was judicially interpreted to require some capacity to survive (*C* v. *S* [1988] QB 135—discussed by Grubb and Pearl, "Protecting the life of the unborn child" (1987) 103 *Law Quarterly Review* 340). However, just how capable of surviving a fetus had to be remained controversial (see *Rance* v. *Mid-Downs HA* [1990] 2 *Med LR* 27). The point will never arise in the future since the 1929 Act does not apply if a doctor performs an abortion in accordance with the 1967 Act

(section 37(4) of the Human Fertilisation and Embryology Act 1990 substituting a new section 5(1) of the Abortion Act 1967). The new legislation is discussed in Grubb, "The New Law of Abortion: Clarification or Ambiguity?" [1991] *Criminal Law Review*.

29. Section 1(1)(*d*) requires "that there is a substantial risk that if the child were born it would suffer from such physical or mental abnormalities as to be seriously handicapped". For a discussion of this ground see Grubb, supra note 24 at 153–4.

30. Section 1(1)(*b*) requires that "termination is necessary to prevent grave permanent injury to the physical or mental health of the pregnant woman".

31. Section 1(1)(*c*) requires that "the continuance of the pregnancy would involve risk to the life of the pregnant woman, greater than if the pregnancy were terminated". Unlike section 1(1)(*b*), this provision requires a comparison of risks between pregnancy and termination. See Grubb supra note 24 on the nature of this exercise.

32. See the discussion by Scowen, "A critique of the Abortion Act amendments?" (1991) 1(2) *Dispatches* 5.

33. It has certainly been assumed that certain body products such as blood (*R* v. *Welsh* [1974] RTR 478) and urine (*R* v. *Rothery* [1976] RTR 550) once separated from the body become property that, as was held in these cases, can be stolen.

34. *Parpalaix v. CECOS and Fédération Française des Centres d'Etude et de Conservation du Sperme* (reproduced in Kennedy and Grubb, *Medical Law* (1989) at 621–2).

35. For an analysis of how English law (prior to the Human Fertilisation and Embryology Act 1990) would deal with this situation see Kennedy and Grubb, ibid. at 622–4.

36. An action might have been brought under the Congenital Disabilities (Civil Liability) Act 1976 by a child born disabled as a result of the negligent damage to gametes during the infertility treatment (see Kennedy and Grubb, supra at 685–7). This has been put beyond doubt by section 44 of the Human Fertilisation and Embryology Act 1990 which inserts into the 1976 Act a new section 1(1A) to cover this situation.

37. (1978) (DC SDNY) (reproduced in Kennedy and Grubb, supra at 656–60).

38. 717 F Supp 421 (ED Va 1989). Discussed by Robertson, "In the beginning: the legal status of early embryos" (1990) 76 *Virginia Law Review* 437 at 461–3.

39. Subject, of course, in England to compliance with the laws relating to testamentary dispositions under the Wills Act 1837.

40. Report of the Committee of Inquiry into Human Fertilisation and Embryology (Cmnd 1314, 1984) at para 10.11.

41. Ibid.

42. See Warnock recommendation supra at para 13.13. It will be a general condition of infertility, storage and research licences granted by the Human Fertilisation and Embryology Authority that "no money or other benefits shall be given or received in respect

of any supply of gametes or embryos unless authorised by directions'' (section 12(e) of the Human Fertilisation and Embryology Act 1990). Presumably, directions will only permit *reasonable expenses* arising from the supply and transportation to be paid as in section 1(3) Human Organs Transplant Act 1989.

43. Supra note 1.
44. For a discussion about the validity of such agreements see Robertson, supra at 463–73.
45. See clause 4(a), (b) and (e) of the specimen consent form in Annex 5 to 1990 Report Of the Interim Licensing Authority.
46. Ibid., clause 4(d).
47. This is consistent with the approach of the Tennessee Court of Appeal in the *Davis* case supra note 4.
48. If sperm or embryo are used after a man's death then he is not in law the father of the child (section 28(6)(b) of Human Fertilisation Act 1990).
49. A similar provision requires the consent of a gamete provider for the use of his or her gametes for treatment services (paragraph 5(1)).
50. Paragraph 7 requires a woman's consent for the use of embryos taken from a woman (by, for example, lavage).
51. A similar provision applies to the storage of gametes when the gamete provider's "effective consent" is required (paragraph 8(1)).
52. Paragraph 8(3) requires the woman's consent where the embryo is taken from her.
53. That it must be written follows from the wording of section 46.
54. Prior to even this, schedule 3 paragraph 3 requires that the gamete providers should "be given a suitable opportunity to receive proper counselling about the implications" of what is to happen and, in addition, should be "provided with such relevant information as is proper".
55. Schedule 3 paragraph 2(1).
56. Ibid., paragraph 8(2).
57. Paragraph 2(1) and (2) respectively. Presumably, if these conditions are unacceptable to the professionals or storage body they will refuse to accept the couple for treatment or as gamete donors.
58. Section 14(4). The period may be shorter if the Authority imposes a shorter period in the storage body's licence. For gametes the maximum storage period is 10 years (section 14(3)), again subject to the terms of the licence.
59. And, of course, gametes.
60. Discussed by Smith, "Australia's frozen orphan embryos: a medical, legal and ethical dilemma" (1985) 24 *Journal of Family Law* 27.
61. See, Infertility (Medical Procedures) Act 1984, section 14—in the absence of any "parental" wishes. For the actual fate of the *Rios* embryos see Kennedy and Grubb, supra at 660.

Maternal-Fetal conflict: reformulating the equation

Ellen J. Stein

Definition

Reproductive medicine is concerned with biological events that occur prior to conception, the conceptual process, gestation and the events that may occur therein, parturition, and the postpartum period. Bioethicists, philosophers and lawyers seem to focus on a particular point in time, or an event that occurs at some point along this biological continuum, such as conception, the termination of a gestation, or the fetal attainment of viability, to establish theoretical positions or to cite legal theory and cases to formulate and justify public policy. As an obstetrician-gynaecologist I am not so concerned with a particular point in time or special event as a marker to construct a medical ethic, as I am with the processes that involve patients and those who provide their medical care.[1]

Maternal-fetal conflict refers to a situation in which a woman disagrees with a plan of medical management or surgical intervention intended by a doctor to benefit her fetus. This type of maternal resistance to professional advice or treatment has been the subject of philosophical, medical, and legal discussion.[2] The definition implies a tension between countervailing interests of mother and fetus, but in reality the conflict may be between the woman and her doctor, and/or other representatives of the medical or legal establishment. The language of adversarial law is rooted in a system of justice which poses rights against obligations. Situations defined as maternal–fetal conflict arise when the "rights" of the fetus are seen to be infringed, or its welfare neglected, by the activities of its mother, who thereby fails to meet her obligations. The initial reality of a conflict between, for instance, hospital personnel on the one hand, and the mother on the other, is thus restated in terms of conflict between the mother and the fetus. This adversarial process encourages the adoption of polarised positions which substitute coercion for explanation, persuasion, negotiation, or compromise.[3] This paper examines the progression of maternal–fetal conflict from the definition of a situation of disagreement to the reality of a crime, in which all parties involved suffer.

Fetal rights: a basis for legal and philosophical controversy

In the UK, the fetus is not a legal entity, i.e. a "person" with defined rights, until it is born and has an independent existence.[4] This is also true in the US with the exception of a very few jurisdictions which have, for some purposes, enacted laws which virtually confer personhood upon the fetus.[5] Nonetheless, both moral and legal claims for the rights of the fetus have been advanced.

Those who uphold such claims argue that, if and when a woman "waives" her right to have an abortion or chooses to carry her fetus to term, she thereby acquires a positive duty to ensure that the fetus will have the healthiest future life possible. Her desires will thus be subordinate to the needs of the fetus.[6]

At the opposite end of this philosophical spectrum is the view that while the occasional rare loss of the life of a fetus or decrease in its eventual quality of life is tragic, neither of these outcomes can justify the abrogation of the mother's fundamental rights to bodily integrity, autonomy, and privacy.[7] The middle ground is characterised by an attempt to use a "balancing" test whereby the relative rights of the mother and the fetus are compared in any given situation. When the risks to the fetus are thought to be significant, in terms of loss of life or eventual severe disability, while the risks to the mother's health or life are relatively lower, the needs of the fetus should prevail, and vice versa.[8] This test is often referred to, in discussions of applied ethics, as the balancing of the prima facie principles of "beneficence" versus "autonomy".[9]

In the US, the primacy of fetal rights is forcefully presented by John Robertson, who argues that "Once [the mother] decides to forgo abortion and the state chooses to protect the fetus, the woman loses the liberty to act in ways that would adversely affect the fetus. Restrictions on pregnancy management may significantly limit a woman's freedom of action and even lead to forcible bodily intrusion to protect the unborn child."[10] He adds, "The mother might also be convicted of child abuse if her action during pregnancy, such as drug and alcohol use, caused an injury to her fetus that lasted after its birth."[11] Robertson's argument relies on: (1) his analysis of Roe v. Wade, the Supreme Court decision that provides constitutional protection to the right to obtain an abortion; (2) analysis of cases in criminal law that might justify conviction for child abuse if prenatal actions cause injury that last after birth, as well as homicide laws that impose liability for prenatal actions that cause death postnatally; and (3) analysis of cases in tort law that require avoidance of actions that will harm fetuses, and provide for damage awards even in cases where the actions have occurred prior to the fetus' attainment of viability.

Oxford lawyer John Eekelaar reasons that once the time has passed when a woman may legally obtain an abortion, "it is morally permissible to draw upon the duties which parents have towards their born children in formulating duties owed to the unborn."[12] He suggests that, amongst other means to ensure that mothers meet their legal duties to their unborn children, orders might be provided for supervision or monitoring of their behaviour after the birth of their children, when their antenatal actions were not thought to be in the unborn child's best interests. In addition, he would restore, in tort law, the right to allow an action by a child for injuries caused to it by its mother before its birth.

Canadian moral philosopher Eike-Henne Kluge proposes an even stronger claim for fetal rights: "once the fetus has passed a certain stage of neurological development it is a person, . . . then the whole issue becomes one of balancing of rights: the right-to-life of the fetal person against the right to autonomy and inviolability of the woman; . . . the fetal right usually wins."[13]

A large body of legal and philosophical literature has arisen in response to Robertson's initial position, much of it expounding a strongly opposing view. Nelson *et al.* have written a paper whose subtitle, "Compelling Each to Live as Seems Good to the Rest", taken from Mill, *On Liberty,* is a hallmark of the approach taken. They argue that "it is far better simply to avoid compelling pregnant women to live as seems good to a particular physician, judge or even to the rest of us, than to force them to sacrifice their wills and their bodies on the altar of someone else's notion of the good".[14] Similar views are expressed by, for example, Gallagher, Rhoden, Annas, Johnsen, and Field.[15] While all of these writers disagree with Robertson's analyses of cases in both tort and criminal law, the most interesting and compelling discussions centre on differing interpretations of constitutional law as it has been interpreted in *Roe* v. *Wade* and other cases.[16]

These cases, heard by the United States Supreme Court, have established the basic framework for constitutional protection of the right to abortion in the US. Using a unified and systematic approach to the problem of ensuring procreative liberty, the Court, eschewing the temptation to decide if or when the fetus acquires rights, and maintaining that the fetus is not a person, examined the relative rights of the state and women in each of the three trimesters of pregnancy. In the first trimester, a woman has an absolute right to abortion, the decision to be reached between her and her physician. In the second trimester, prior to the attainment of viability of the fetus, a woman has the right to abortion subject only to regulations proposed by the state that would serve to protect the health interests of the mother. In the third trimester, after attainment of viability of the fetus, abortion is prohibited, except to preserve the health or life of the mother, because of the "state's compelling interest in protecting potential life". Attempts in state law to compel methods of abortion that would enhance the possibility of fetal survival have been rebuffed by the Court on grounds that the mother's health interests are paramount. Gallagher summarises the position relating to maternal–fetal conflict: "A pregnant woman carries with her all the common dignities and rights accorded by the law. In a disagreement with her care giver during the course of her medical treatment, she may assert not only the generally available rights of bodily integrity, self-determination, and conscientious liberty, but those constitutional protections particular to her situation: the right of procreative and familial decision making."[17]

A similarly strong view of the pregnant woman's rights in law in the UK is expressed by Diana Brahams, who concludes a recent "Medicine and the Law" column on enforced caesarean sections in the US as follows: "In British Law, where there is a conflict between the interests of the fetus and the mother, the interests and wishes of the mother must prevail."[18] She is joined by Derek Morgan, whose final comment on a British attempt to make an unborn child a ward of court in *Re F* (*in utero*) posits [that] "Even if there may be a course to be set between the Scylla of treating women as foetal containers and the Charybdis of regarding their foetuses as uterine cargo, the price which we must be prepared to pay for protecting the integrity and autonomy of *all* competent adults is the rare, occasional risk of death or serious injury to an unborn foetus."[19]

The middle ground of this moral and legal philosophical spectrum is, in some ways, the most difficult to define, delineate, and defend. Engelhardt, Blank, and Noble-Allgire provide theses from medical, philosophical, and legal points of view.[20] Taken as a whole, this position grants the fundamental importance of autonomy, privacy, and bodily integrity to women, but considers the rights of a fetus, when viable and meant by the mother to be brought to term, to be of equal importance if its well-being is significantly threatened. The problem these theorists face is deciding, in each and every case, what balance may be most equitably struck. This position reflects, of course, the problems that practising obstetricians face every day.

The British equivalent of "middle-ground" theorists, such as Kennedy, Bainham, and Fortin, also propose a balancing test approach, where the liberty interests of the mother are weighed against the putative rights of the unborn child.[21] In the UK, however, these arguments are cast against the light of an entirely different abortion law.

Unlike abortion legislation in the US, obtaining an abortion in the UK, until April 1991, depended on the interplay between two Acts, the Abortion Act 1967 and the Infant Life (Preservation) Act 1929. The Abortion Act provided that a doctor was free to terminate a pregnancy, with the intention of killing a fetus, if two registered medical practitioners were of the opinion, in good faith, that the continuance of the pregnancy would involve risk to the life of the pregnant woman, or risk of injury to the physical or mental health of the pregnant woman or any existing children of her family, greater than if the pregnancy were terminated; or that there was a substantial risk that if the child were born it would suffer from such physical or mental abnormalities as to be seriously handicapped.

The Act specifically stated that nothing within it would affect the Infant Life (Preservation) Act 1929, which states that any person, with intent to destroy the life of a child capable of being born alive, is guilty of child destruction, provided that the act which caused the death of the child was not done in good faith for the purpose only of preserving the life of the mother.[22]

These Acts, then, were passed to protect medical practitioners primarily, and give patients access to abortion through the medical opinion of professionals. There was no hint of shared decision-making between patient and doctor, although in practice that may indeed have taken place. Nor was there discussion of the "state's compelling interest in protecting life" after viability, although in practice, "capable of being born alive" was taken to coincide with viability. In these Acts and associated tort and criminal law, there was no question of whether the fetus could be a "person" before birth; it was not.

The Human Fertilisation and Embryology Act 1990, along with amendments to The Abortion Act 1967, was enacted in November 1990 and the abortion amendments took effect on 1 April 1991. The grounds for medical termination of pregnancy were not substantially changed, but were specifically restricted to pregnancies not exceeding the 24th week if "the continuance of the pregnancy would involve risk, greater than if the pregnancy were terminated, of injury to the physical or mental health of the pregnant woman or any existing children of her family".[23] The other grounds for termination contained in the new section 1(1) of the 1967 Act are prevention of "grave permanent injury to the physical or mental health of the pregnant woman", "risk to the life of the pregnant woman", or "substantial risk that if the child were born it would suffer from such physical or mental abnormalities as to be seriously handicapped". These grounds are specifically exempted from the 24 week time limit. This was accomplished by "unlinking" the Abortion Act 1967 from the Infant Life (Preservation) Act 1929. The new section 5(1) of the 1967 Act provides that "No offence under the Infant Life (Preservation) Act 1929 shall be committed by a registered medical practitioner who terminates a pregnancy in accordance with the provisions of this Act".[24]

Against this recent change in legal background, the balancing equations of the British legal philosophers take on unusual importance. Kennedy, while commending a "calculus" to compare the relative needs of pregnant women and their fetuses, concludes that it would not serve the interests of public policy to enact enforcing legislation.[25] Bainham, on the other hand, states that a proper balance between the interests of the mother and those of the unborn child is required, and that "there appears to be no reason why wardship [of the unborn child] could not be utilised for this kind of exercise".[26] Fortin, in a novel suggestion intended to achieve legal coherence, proposes that abortions be limited to 10 weeks' gestation, and experimentation on human embryos extended to 10 weeks, on the basis of Lockwood's concept that the fetus becomes a "human being" at that time, having achieved sufficient neurological development to meet that criterion.[27]

Medical opinion[28] on changes in the law on abortion has centred on the issue of "seriously handicapped" fetuses, as it is in this arena that medical practice might be most likely to change. Grave maternal illness as a medical indication for termination of pregnancies beyond 24 weeks has never posed an ethical dilemma for doctors, as the intention has never been to destroy the life of the fetus but rather to save the life of the mother, and in so doing, enhance the survival of the infant as well. On the other hand, an ethical "balancing act" applied in the cases of affected fetuses will involve consideration of the severity of handicap, gestational age at time of diagnosis, the infant's life expectancy, the mother's past obstetric history and desires, and the obstetrician's willingness to be guided by all or any of these matters.

After the amendments to the 1967 Act, the law in the UK relating to late termination of pregnancies is far more liberal than that in America. There, fetal handicap is not given consideration for termination of pregnancy beyond attainment of "viability". In the words of a consultant obstetrician in Scotland, "Liberalization of the law will probably not be used extensively to increase the number of late terminations. Nevertheless, the knowledge that a carefully considered, well documented termination for fetal malformation diagnosed after 24 weeks will fall within the scope of the abortion legislation is welcome."[29]

While the new law provides for flexibility in medical treatment of individual cases, it may encourage legal intervention parallel to the US practice of balancing the rights of the fetus versus those of the mother.

Involvement of the courts in maternal-fetal conflict

The fetus cannot speak for itself; its "interests", in medical, moral, and legal terms, must be both presented and represented by third parties. Presently, in situations involving maternal-fetal conflict in the US, a third party, usually but not always a doctor, hospital representative, or social worker, requests a court order to enforce medical care such as caesarean section, intrauterine transfusion, or hospital detention when the mother does not wish such care. Such requests are motivated by a desire to avert possible harm to the fetus when there is medical uncertainty, or intensive use of medical technology is available. Fear of malpractice liability may be a consideration, as may other factors, cognitive and emotive, conscious and unconscious.[30]

The practice of requesting court orders to ensure maternal compliance with medical decisions was first brought to wide attention by George Annas in 1982, when he published a seminal article on forced caesarean sections. In that paper, he described two cases which have been cited subsequently in numerous legal and philosophical discussions to support opposing points of view.[31] In addition to raising important questions on the state of the law, the role of the judiciary in labour room disputes, and what position physicians and hospitals should take when confronted with women who refuse caesarean section against medical advice, his concerns actually presaged future events. One specific question raised by Annas was whether these cases could "be distinguished from other medical interventions, including fetal surgery, if and when it becomes accepted medical procedure, or would women be forced to consent to these as well? And if one can lawfully force surgery, one should certainly be able to restrain the liberty of a woman for the sake of her fetus, e.g., by confining her during all or part of her pregnancy."[32]

In 1985, Chervenak and McCullough published a paper on perinatal ethics in the official journal of the American College of Obstetricians and Gynecologists (ACOG) in which they offered "a practical method of analysis of obligations to mother and fetus''. Using a scheme which weighed the best interests of the mother against the best interests of the fetus, they considered each of these best interests in the light of the physician's "autonomy-based" and "beneficence-based" obligations towards the mother, and the "beneficence-based" obligations of both mother and physician towards the fetus. For each of these categories of moral obligation, they considered the possible conflicts that might arise, and the appropriate moral responses that physicians might have to consider. In several cases, they concluded that beneficence-based obligations should override autonomy-based obligations, requiring the doctor to take actions to which the mother may not agree. While they stated that remedies short of legal action such as vigorous persuasion "involve fewer negative consequences for the physician–patient relationship and maternal–infant bonding", sometimes "A more coercive approach, e.g. threatening to seek or seeking a court order, may be morally justifiable."[33]

While it is difficult to know what effect articles like these actually have on the behaviour of obstetricians, the portents for the future raised by Annas were reflected five years later in an article by Kolder *et al.* They reported, in a retrospective survey of 61 heads of fellowship programmes in maternal–fetal medicine in the US, that, during the previous five years, 21 court orders for caesarean section, hospital detentions, and intrauterine transfusions had been sought. In 86 per cent of those requested, the orders were obtained; 88 per cent of these orders were received within six hours. Most importantly, although the responses to the opinion portion of the survey were sharply divided, 47 per cent of programme heads thought that "the precedent set by the courts in cases requiring emergency caesarean sections for the sake of the fetus should be extended to include *other procedures that are potentially lifesaving for the fetus, such as intrauterine transfusion, as these procedures come to represent the standard of care"* (emphasis added).[34] The authors emphasise that the common element in these cases is an adversarial contest between the rights of the mother and those of the fetus, towards whom she has responsibilities.

In 1987, the Committee on Ethics of the American College of Obstetricians and Gynecologists was prompted by concern at the increasing use of court orders in the practice of obstetrics to state that "The use of the courts to resolve [these] conflicts is almost never warranted".[35] Further, in 1989, ACOG produced a Technical Bulletin, "Ethical decision-making in obstetrics and gynecology" stating: "Although it may be agreed that a pregnant woman has fundamental obligations toward her fetus, no other party, including the state, should override her autonomy in order to enforce those obligations."[36]

Court-ordered interventions in obstetrical care have not been reported in the UK, although there have been several attempts in law to achieve them. In *Re F (in utero)*, in 1988, an English court denied a petition to ward an unborn child so that the mother could be detained and antenatal care enforced against her will on the grounds that it represented an unwarranted infringement of her liberty.[37]

Though maternal–fetal conflict, logically defined, could be said to occur only between a wanted fetus and its mother, the concept has been extended to cover other situations. An attempt in *C v. S* was made to seek a court order to prevent the termination of a fetus of less than 28 weeks' gestation.[38] The attempt failed in law, although in this instance the termination did not take place. The case of *D (a minor) v. Berks CC* and others[39] was contested until it reached the House of Lords. That body upheld a juvenile court order, which, under the Children and Young Persons Act 1969, committed the newborn child of a woman who had taken drugs during pregnancy to the care and control of the local authority. It was felt that the mother had endangered the child's proper development or health by failing to cooperate fully with medical advice during pregnancy. This may be seen as an extension of the concept of maternal–fetal conflict *in retrospect*, as the evidence for neglect of the child applied to the time when the child was *in utero*. There was no cause to believe that the mother would neglect the child in the same way, in the future, by administering drugs to it. It might also be classified as a case of "fetal abuse", a term coming into increasing usage in the US.

A new continuum: from maternal–fetal conflict to fetal abuse

In 1987, the same year as the Kolder survey, one of the most notorious cases of maternal–fetal conflict in the US, *In re AC*, began to evolve. In Washington, DC in 1987, a hospital sought a declaratory order to perform a caesarean section on a woman terminally ill with cancer who was 26 weeks pregnant. The patient had previously agreed to treatment that would prolong her life so as to increase the fetus' chance of healthy survival, hoping to reach a gestational age of 28 weeks. However, she refused a caesarean delivery for the sake of the fetus at 26 weeks, when a neonatologist estimated fetal viability at 50–60 per cent with a less than 20 per cent risk of serious handicap. In spite of family members' and clinicians' agreement with her refusal, the Superior Court entered an order permitting the caesarean section. On appeal, motion for stay was denied by the Court of Appeals. The surgery was performed: the premature infant died within two hours, the mother within two days. The case was decided on the basis "that mother's penumbral privacy right against bodily intrusion was properly subordinated to interests of unborn child and state".[40] Since, according to the Court, the "interests of unborn child and state" required intrusion into (or obligation upon) the body of the mother, the corresponding right had then to be ascribed to her fetus.

The decision was vacated on 18 March 1988, in response to petition by the appellants and 39 *amici curiae*, including ACOG and the American Medical Association. However, it remained a standing precedent until 26 April 1990, when the Court, after an *en banc* rehearing, published its new decision.[41]

Judge Terry's opinion, on behalf of the Court (with one judge dissenting in part), was a model in law for the right to bodily integrity and the right of a person's wishes regarding medical treatment, whether they are competent or incompetent, to be respected. He held that "in virtually all cases the question of what is to be done is to be decided by the patient—the pregnant woman—on behalf of herself and the fetus". The trial judge was not to engage in a "balancing" exercise, weighing the interests of the patient and the interests of the fetus. The primacy of the woman's rights was found to be supported by both common law and the Constitution. Moreover, if the patient was found to be incompetent, the doctrine of "substituted judgment" was to be used in reaching a decision, to determine what the patient *herself* would have wanted. The problem with the decision lies not in what was found, but in the narrowness of its application. Judge Terry specifically refused to extend the opinion to the District of Columbia case of *In re Madyun*[42] where caesarean section had been ordered when the mother was healthy and the baby was at term, the procedure had been refused on religious grounds, and it had been decided by medical staff that the procedure would benefit both the mother and the baby. He also would not consider the implications in this decision for the performance of less invasive procedures, such as ultrasound examination or transfusions.

Professor Robertson has recently modified his original position to the extent that, while still maintaining the constitutional validity of "pre-birth seizures", he now regards "post-birth sanctions" as being sounder health policy.[43] Courts and legislatures are increasingly making use of such sanctions in attempting to influence reproductive outcome by threat of eventual criminal prosecution for what is now termed "fetal abuse". Two cases presently in the Florida court system are likely to rival *In re AC* in notoriety. One involves a woman who was convicted on 13 July 1989 for "delivering" a cocaine derivative through the umbilical cord to two babies after their births but before the cords were clamped. Although neither child is addicted nor disabled, the mother was sentenced to 200 hours of community service and probation for 14 years, during which she must, in addition to other requirements, submit to any physical examinations and random searches of her belongings, and remain employed. The state learned of her addiction to cocaine because she had confided in her obstetrician. The conviction has recently been upheld on appeal. In a similar case, another mother was, in addition, charged with contributing to the delinquency or dependency of a minor.[44]

Research and health policy

Research in the area of maternal–fetal conflict and fetal abuse is still scant and imperfect, but certain trends are becoming apparent. In the Kolder survey, demographic data on the patients were reported; they suggested that court-ordered obstetrical interventions occur predominantly in patients who are disadvantaged, from a minority, or non-English speaking.[45] Unfortunately, the methodology of the survey was both retrospective and uncontrolled. Therefore, while the conclusions on patient characteristics may be true, they have yet to be proven. However, the point that the authors make is well taken:

professionals are allowed the freedom perhaps to make mistakes of judgment in overusing technology under the protective umbrella of court orders, but patients are denied the opportunity to make the opposite choice.

To this point, there are, as yet, no studies of morbidity and mortality that compare cases in which court orders have been granted and implemented with those which were requested and denied, or not implemented. Jordan and Irwin have written several articles on the problem of court-ordered caesarean sections. Their most recent reports six cases in which court orders were sought and obtained for caesarean section between 1979 and 1986. Of these, two resulted in caesarean section, one delivery method was unknown, and three had vaginal deliveries (one at another hospital, one while legal proceedings were ongoing at the same hospital, and one at the same hospital, after a repeat sonogram showed the placenta praevia had "migrated").[46] A morbidity and mortality outcome study is, therefore, clearly warranted.

In a careful, controlled study, Dr M.L. Poland looked for differences between patients with good and poor antenatal clinic attendance records. All the patients were equally economically disadvantaged and practically all were from a minority group. Patients who attended poorly or not at all ("walk-ins" to the labour and delivery suite) were "older, had more children, were at high risk for complication, experienced shorter pregnancies and produced smaller babies".[47] They also depended less on information and advice from written materials and professionals, assigned a lower value to prenatal care, feared doctors more, and had beliefs about risk factors that were often at variance with standard medical practice. In other words, the women at highest risk for problems perceived them least accurately, at least from a medical point of view.

These data, though far from definitive, indicate the futility of coercion, whether by "pre-birth seizure" or by "post-birth sanction", on the women who need the most help. Such proceedings, whether civil or criminal, are unlikely to deter addiction to tobacco, alcohol or drugs. Poland's findings therefore support those policy makers who favour non-interventionist and non-sanctionary policies and advocate programmes of education and rehabilitation.

A recent article, "The prevalence of illicit-drug or alcohol use during pregnancy and discrepancies in mandatory reporting in Pinellas County, Florida'',[48] reported that, among 715 pregnant women anonymously screened for the presence of alcohol, opiates, cocaine and cannabinoids in urine collected at the first prenatal visit, the prevalence of a positive result on the toxicological tests was 14.8 per cent. Of the women, 380 had enrolled at five public health clinics; 335 enrolled at any of 12 private obstetrical offices in the county. These results were collected over a six month period. Florida is one of the states that require that mothers known to have used alcohol or illicit drugs during pregnancy be reported to health authorities. The regulations require reporting when there is an "admission by the mother of drug use during pregnancy, or a positive maternal drug screen during pregnancy or the early postpartum period, or a positive newborn drug screen. Documentation of maternal drug abuse or drug addiction is not necessary for an infant to be included under the mandatory-reporting regulation. Thus, the regulations focus on the infant's exposure, not the mother's pattern of drug or alcohol use."[49]

The researchers found little objective difference in prevalence of drug exposure between the women seen at the public clinics (16.3 per cent) and those seen at the private offices (13.1 per cent). They found no significant difference between white women (15.4 per cent) and black women (14.1 per cent). However, over the same period of time as the urine collection, 133 women were reported after delivery for substance abuse during pregnancy. "Despite the similar rates of substance abuse among black and white women in the study, black women were reported at approximately 10 times the rate for white women (P<0.0001), and poor women were more likely than others to be reported."[50] The authors conclude that use of illicit drugs is common among pregnant women, and that if "legally mandated reporting is to be free of racial or economic bias, it must be based on objective medical criteria."[51]

The two cases presently before the Florida court system involving "fetal abuse" by "delivery of cocaine" have criminalised two mothers who happen to be black. In the light of the above research, it would appear that this approach is unjust, unwise, and discriminatory. The conceptual slope from maternal–fetal conflict to fetal abuse has proved slippery indeed; the implications for appropriate health policy as well as the proper practice of everyday obstetric medicine are grave. Our legal and medical policies should be formulated more on the basis of sound empirical data and less on the basis of intellectually compelling but unscientifically grounded moral philosophies. How else shall we maintain the maxim that "Medicine is the most humane of sciences, the most empiric of arts, and the most scientific of humanities"?[52]

Notes and references

1. E. Stein and C. Redman, "Decision making in difficult pregnancies", in 49th proceedings Soc. App. Anth. 1990: *Assembling Knowledge to Address Human Problems.* E. Stein and C. Redman, "Maternal-fetal conflict: A definition (1990) 58 *Medico-Legal Journal* 230–5.
2. M. Mahowald, "Beyond abortion: refusal of caesarean section" *Bioethics* (1989) 3 106–21. R. H. Blank, "Emerging notions of women's rights and responsibilities during gestation" (1986) 7 *Journal of Legal Medicine* 441–69. L. J. Nelson and N. Milliken, "Compelled medical treatment of pregnant women" (1988) 259 *Journal of the American Medical Association* 1060–6. V. Kolder, J. Gallagher and M. Parsons, "Court-ordered obstetrical interventions" (1987) 316 *New England Journal of Medicine* 1192–6. G. Annas, "The impact of medical technology on the pregnant woman's right to privacy" (1987) 13 *American Journal of Law and Medicine* 213–32. J. Robertson, "Gestational burdens and fetal status: justifying Roe v. Wade" (1987) 13 *American Journal of Law and Medicine* 189–212. D. Brahams, "Enforced caesarean section: a US appeal" (1990) 335 *Lancet* 1270. D. Morgan, "*Re F (in utero)*" (1988) *Journal of Social Welfare Law* 197–203.
3. Stein and Redman, op. cit. note 1.
4. *C* v. *S* [1988] QB 135 (QBD and CA).
5. *Webster* v. *Reproductive Health Services* (1989) 57 LW 5023. *Davis* v. *Davis* (1989) 15 FLR 2097 (Tenn Cir Ct Blount Cty).
6. J. Eekelaar, "Does a mother have legal duties to her unborn child?" P. A. Byrne ed., *Health, Rights and Resources,* (Oxford: Kings' Fund/OUP 1988) pp. 55–75. E-H. Kluge, "When caesarean section operations imposed by a court are justified" (1988) 14 *Journal of Medical Ethics* 206–211. J. Robertson, "Procreative liberty and the control of conception, pregnancy, and childbirth" (1983) 69 *Virginia Law Review* 405–464.
7. J. Gallagher, "Prenatal invasions and interventions: what's wrong with fetal rights" (1987) 10 *Harvard Women's Law Journal* 9–58. N. K. Rhoden, "Cesareans and samaritans" (1987) 15 *Law Medicine and Health Care* 118–25. L. Nelson, B. Buggy and C. Weil, "Forced medical treatment of pregnant women; 'Compelling each to live as seems good to the rest'" (1986) 37 *Hastings Law Journal* 703–63.
8. A. Nobile-Allgire, "Court-ordered cesarean sections: A judicial

106 CHALLENGES IN MEDICAL CARE

standard for resolving the conflict between fetal interests and maternal rights" (1989) 10 *Journal of Legal Medicine* 211-49. R. H. Blank, "Emerging notions of women's rights and responsibilities during gestation" (1986) 7 *Journal of Legal Medicine* 441-69.

9. T. Beauchamp and J. Childress, *Principles of Biomedical Ethics* (New York: Oxford University Press, 1989).
10. J. Robertson, "Procreative liberty and the control of conception, pregnancy, and childbirth" (1983) 69 *Virginia Law Review* 405-64 at p.437.
11. Ibid. at p.439.
12. Eekelaar, op. cit. at p.65.
13. Kluge, op. cit. at p.206.
14. Nelson, Buggy, Weil, op. cit. at p.763.
15. Gallagher, op. cit., Rhoden, op. cit., Annas, op. cit. D. Johnsen, "The creation of fetal rights: conflicts with women's constitutional rights to liberty, privacy and equal protection" (1986) 95 *Yale Law Journal* 599-625. M. Field, "Controlling the woman to protect the fetus (1989) 17 *Law, Medicine and Health Care* 114-29.
16. *Roe v. Wade* 410 U.S. 113 (1973). Also, *Doe v. Bolton* 410 U.S. 179 (1973); *Coluatti v. Franklin* 439 U.S. 379, 394 (1979); *City of Akron v. Akron Center for Reproductive Health* 462 U.S. 416 (1983); *American College of Obstetricians & Gynecologists v. Thornburgh* 737 F. 2d 283, 299 (3d Cir. 1984) *aff'd,* 106 S. Ct. 2106 (1986).
17. Gallagher, op. cit. at p.54.
18. Brahams, op. cit.
19. Morgan, op. cit. at p.203, partially citing W. Mecker, in (1987) 317 *New England Journal of Medicine* at p.1224.
20. H. T. Engelhardt, "Current controversies in obstetrics: wrongful life and forced fetal surgical procedures" (1985) 151 *American Journal of Obstetrics and Gynecology* 313-18. Blank, op. cit. Noble-Allgire, op. cit.
21. I. Kennedy, "A woman and her unborn child: rights and responsibilities" in P. Byrne, ed., *Ethics and Law in Health Care and Research,* (Chichester: John Wiley, 1990) pp.161-186. A. Bainham, "Wardship: effect and uses Re F (in utero)" (1988) 138 *New Law Journal* 123-4. J. Fortin, "Legal protection for the unborn child" (1988) 51 *Modern Law Review* 54-83.
22. P. D. G. Skegg, *Law, Ethics, and Medicine,* (Oxford: Clarendon Press 1988) chapter 1.
23. Human Fertilisation and Embryology Act 1990 Section 37(1)(*a*) amending Abortion Act 1967, section 1(1).
24. Effected by ibid., section 37(1)(4).
25. Kennedy, op. cit.
26. Bainham, op. cit. at p.124.
27. Fortin, op. cit. at p.58. This point is particularly unconvincing from an embryological point of view. See H. Risemberg, a neonatologist, who explains that in the development of the cerebral cortex, neuronal migration of millions of cells may be detected as early as the second month and beyond the fifth month of gestation. This fact

alone would make it presumptuous to designate *one moment*, such as at 10 weeks in fetal development, when neurological development could be said to represent a mental status equivalent to that of a "human being". In "Fetal neglect and abuse" (1989) *New York State Journal of Medicine* (March) 148–51, at p.149.

28. M. H. Hall, "Changes in the law on abortion" (1990) 331 *British Medical Journal* 1109–10.
29. Ibid. at p.1110.
30. Stein and Redman, op. cit. note 1.
31. G. Annas, "Forced cesarean sections: the most unkindest cut of all" (1982) 12 *Hastings Center Report* (3) 16–17, 45. The cases cited were: *Jefferson* v. *Griffin Spalding Co. Hospital Authority* 274 S.E. 2d 457 (1981) and *Raleigh Fitkin-Paul Morgan Memorial Hospital* v. *Anderson* 201 A. 2d 537, 538 (N.J. 1964). These cases, represent, in law, the state's finding that obstetrical interventions may be ordered over patients' objections. Yet in neither case was the intervention actually carried out: in the first the mother had a normal vaginal delivery after a caesarean section had been ordered; in the second, the mother avoided an ordered blood transfusion by leaving the hospital, and subsequently had a normal birth without transfusion. The cases are used as bases for argument from the points of view of two differing realities: that of (1) the law, and (2) outcomes as actual medical events.
32. Ibid. at p.45.
33. F. Chervenak and L. McCullough, "Perinatal ethics: a practical method of analysis of obligations to mother and fetus" (1985) 66 *Obstetrics and Gynecology* 442–446, at p.445.
34. Kolder, op. cit. at p.1193.
35. ACOG Committee Opinion. Patient choice: maternal–fetal conflict. October 1987; 55.
36. ACOG Technical Bulletin. "Ethical decision-making in obstetrics and gynecology", November 1989; 136, at p.4.
37. *Re F* (*in utero*) [1988] 2 All ER 193.
38. *C* v. *S* (supra note 4).
39. *D* v. *Berkshire County Council* [1987] 1 All ER 20.
40. *In re AC* 533 A. 2d 611 (DC App 1987) at 611.
41. *In re AC* 573 A. 2d 1235 (DC App *en banc*) (1990).
42. *In re Madyun* 114 Daily Wash. L. Reptr. 2233 (D.C. Super. Ct. July 26, 1986).
43. J. Robertson, "Fetal abuse" (1989) 75 *American Bar Association Journal* 38–9. See also: S. Balisy, "Maternal substance abuse: the need to provide legal protection for the fetus" (1987) 60 *Southern California Law Review* 1209–38; M. Shaw, "Conditional prospective rights of the fetus" (1984) 5 *Journal of Legal Medicine* 63.
44. L. Gostin, "An ASLM briefing: women and health" (1990) 3 *American Society of Law and Medicine Briefings* 1,5, citing unpublished cases.
45. Kolder, op. cit. at p.1195.

46. B. Jordan and S. L. Irwin, "The ultimate failure: court-ordered cesarean section", in L. M. Whiteford and M. L. Poland eds, *New Approaches to Human Reproduction* (Boulder and London: Westview Press, 1989) pp.13–24.

47. M. Poland, "Ethical issues in the delivery of quality care to pregnant indident women", in Whiteford and Poland, ibid.: 42–50, p.44.

48. I. Chasnoff, H. Landress and M. Barrett, "The prevalence of illicit-drug or alcohol use during pregnancy and discrepancies in mandatory reporting in Pinellas County, Florida" (1990) 322 *New England Journal of Medicine* 1202–6.

49. Ibid. at p.1203.

50. Ibid. at p.1202.

51. Ibid.

52. E. Pellegrino, "The most humane science: Some notes on liberal education in medicine and the university", The Sixth Sanger Lecture, *Bulletin*, Medical College of Virginia, Volume LXVII(4), p.13.

Medical accountability: a background paper

Margaret Stacey

This paper will discuss the issues raised by the General Medical Council's (GMC) recent proposals about machinery to deal with incompetent doctors and attempt to put these proposals in the more general context of how doctors should be held to account.[1]

Nature of accountability

As Day and Klein[2] have indicated, the notion of accountability is an ancient one with a long career and has had different implications over time. Nowadays as I understand it (with the aid of the OED), to be accountable is in essence to be bound to give account and is the same as to be responsible—for things or to people or more abstractly. In accountability there is a sense of necessary requirement—one is bound to give account of one's action, to be answerable. So how and in what way are contemporary medical practitioners held to account?

But what exactly is medical accountability? There are so many ways in which a doctor may be held to account for his/her actions: for clinical actions to individual patients and, in medical audit, to colleagues; by law in terms of obligations to patient or employer; to the profession for her/his behaviour; to employers for the money spent and the priorities adopted in treatments; to the state in relation to contracts. Furthermore, as a collectivity the profession is held to account to the public at large for the quality of medical care in general and in particular.

There is a remarkable array in present day Britain of procedures involving one or other of these kinds of accountability. The procedures may be divided into four types:

1. professional, based on self-regulation;
2. NHS: disciplinary and to handle complaints;
3. Parliamentary;
4. legal.

None of the procedures taken singly nor the total array is felt to be altogether satisfactory. Discontent is felt (albeit for different reasons) by everybody who becomes involved one way or another with medical accountability, be they practitioners in the medical or associated professions, patients or their representatives, health service managers and administrators, policy makers or governments.

Origins of the multiple modes of regulation

This disparate array has two main roots. The first lies in the concept of profession development in the 19th century by a body of practitioners engaged in the one-to-one treatment of individual patients.[3] The second derives from the developing responsibilities felt by governments to ensure the provision of adequate medical care for its citizens. The institutions and practices which have resulted have a variety of aims, some not being concerned with accountability alone, others with accountability in one sense but not, or only secondarily, in another.

Professional origins

The General Medical Council (GMC), founded in 1858 by Act of Parliament as the statutory body responsible for the regulation of the medical profession, has a central place. The GMC embodies the crucial concept of professional self-regulation which Merrison saw "as a contract between public and profession, by which the public go to the profession for medical treatment because the profession has made sure it will provide satisfactory treatment".[4]

Medical and other healing practices have always been regulated in some way. The Church, the Colleges (some of which in time became Royal Colleges and flourish today), other bodies (of which the Society of Apothecaries survives) and the Universities have all at one time or another been involved in the regulation of practice. The Royal Colleges, the Faculties and the Universities continue to play important regulatory roles, as do the defence societies and the British Medical Association (BMA) which, while essentially being a trade union, does seek to enhance professional standards of practice and behaviour. However, it was the General Medical Council which laid the basis for our contemporary unified medical profession. Through it the primacy of biomedicine (as it may best be referred to nowadays) over all other healing modes was established. The Council played an important role in facilitating the high status which medicine gradually achieved through the 19th century and which it still enjoys.

Origins in state health care

A second set of arrangements, which developed later, derives from the state's involvement in providing appropriate medical care for its citizens and its ultimate responsibility for the expenditure of public money. In this way the state's interest in medical practitioners working for the NHS is different from its interest in the regulation of the profession as such—which it ceded in 1858 to the GMC—and has led to a different set of regulatory procedures.

Because of the different employment arrangements for hospital doctors and general practitioners, their mode of accountability to the NHS has been, and remains, different. With regard to general practitioners—and others like them who work as independent practitioners under contract to the state—the state's concern, which dates back to the National Health Insurance Act of 1911, is that they fulfil their contracts. These practitioners are answerable for doing properly what they have contracted to do, but, in this context, answerable for that only. Any accountability to the state (through the—now—Family Health Services Authority procedures) for the treatment, non-treatment or mistreatment of patients emerged as a secondary consequence of the accountability for fulfilling the contracts. Like all others, family practitioners are also accountable to the

GMC for their proper professional conduct and as citizens to the law courts.

With regard to those in NHS hospital practice, initially the Ministry of Health (as it then was) thought that the mode of accountability which applied to civil servants would be appropriate, since doctors are employed in hospitals on a salary basis. Later it became obvious that the nature of hospital medicine was such that purpose-built arrangements would be needed. The result is that we now have two procedures: the disciplinary proceedings for medical staffs (under Government Circular HM(61)112) and the complaints machinery for aggrieved patients or their representatives (under Government Circular HC(88)37). The latter is, relatively, a latecomer, arriving 10 years after the Davies Committee on Hospital Complaints Procedures[5] had indicated machinery was necessary, delay having been created on the medical side.

The procedures

Professional self-regulation

With regard to accountability within the profession exercised on behalf of the profession and the public, two aspects are of particular importance. The first is medical audit; the second the role of the GMC.

1. Medical audit   Medical audit, under a variety of names, has been around for a long time[6] particularly in the US. In the UK the Confidential Enquiry into Maternal Deaths, set up in the 1930s by the Royal College of Obstetrics and Gynaecology (RCOG), is probably the earliest systematic peer review of outcome in clinical practice. The Association of Anaesthetists of Great Britain commissioned an enquiry into anaesthetic deaths in the 1950s and subsequently they have undertaken a further two. There have been various enquiries into surgical performance and outcome, but nothing on the scale of the work of the anaesthetists or the RCOG. The Confidential Enquiry into Perioperative Deaths (CEPOD) which covers anaesthesia and surgery is a recent development aimed at filling this gap.[7] This covered three regions only and has now been succeeded by the National Confidential Enquiry into Perioperative Deaths

(NCEPOD).[8] There have also been audits in the medical arena.[9] These examples, although important, have been somewhat scattered. Wilmot[10] has summarised methods used for medical audit in primary care citing particularly the Royal College of General Practitioners (RCGP) working party reports.[11]

Nevertheless, medical audit has not hitherto been widely, systematically or continuously applied to the process and outcomes of treatment. Medical audit, however, seems likely to be treated a great deal more seriously than hitherto since its importance was stressed in the Government's White Paper *Working for Patients*[12] in January 1989, and in March 1989 was the subject of a report from the Royal College of Physicians of London and of guidance from the Royal College of Surgeons of England.[13] The Royal College of Physicians have not only come out in favour of audit, but have made it clear that approval for hospital training posts may be withheld if adequate medical audit meetings are not conducted. This also seems to be implied in the Surgeons' guidelines.

So far as the Royal College of Physicians is concerned medical audit is primarily a mechanism for

— assessing and improving the quality of patient care;
— enhancing medical education by promoting discussion between colleagues about practice;
— identifying ways of improving the efficiency of clinical care.

The College also stresses the equivalent importance in medical audit of

— structure, e.g. the quantity and type of resources,
— process—what was done to the patient,
— and outcome—in terms such as duration of survival, quality of life, residual disability.

The Physicians insist on the importance of the cycle of audit which includes

— standard setting,
— observing and comparing practice against standards implementing change.

As McKee, Lauglo and Lessof stress: ''To be meaningful audit procedures must complete this cycle.''[14]

Medical practitioners see medical audit as an essentially profession-led activity. They draw a clear distinction between clinical audit to improve patient care and managerial audit aimed at reducing costs.[15] What makes medical audit different from "grand rounds" or other forms of staff meeting and discussion is its systematic nature: the regularity of meetings, the use of numerate records and analyses, and the definitive inclusion of patient outcome. Hitherto, with the honourable exceptions mentioned, stress in medical self-regulation has tended to be on process rather than on outcome.

2. The General Medical Council The single most important institution of professional self-regulation is, of course, the General Medical Council. Its disciplinary procedures and the way they are operated have influence well beyond the confines of the Council chamber and the particular cases dealt with there. The Council may not have been "formed to be a parliament for making professional laws or a union for protecting professional interests",[16] but by virtue of its statutory function as regulator of the profession, the pronouncements and behaviour of the GMC do set the tone for the entire profession.

The GMC's main regulatory instrument is the Register of qualified medical practitioners. "The maintenance of a register of the competent is fundamental to the regulation of a profession."[17] This comprises two duties: ensuring that those admitted to the register are competent, and removing those unfit to practice.[18] The GMC has come in for criticism for paying insufficient attention to the latter so far as clinical competence is concerned.[19]

In 1987 the GMC "set up a working party on the Council's disciplinary procedures in response to allegations of failure to provide a good standard of medical care", intending to

> examine the issue of the establishment of competence procedures, under its jurisdiction, to help it respond to complaints about standards of care provided by doctors which appear to arise from failures of competence.[20]

This working party reported in May 1989.[21] It made some 16 recommendations in all; in what follows I have grouped them somewhat differently from the way the working party did.

The most innovatory proposal is that there should be new procedures established to deal with doctors alleged to be incompetent, not all within the Council; some should take place at local level. The Council will formulate such proposals and invite the profession to discuss them; the suggested procedures will take account of arrangements for medical audit in the NHS and bear in mind doctors not covered by these procedures. The working party reiterated the distinction which has in the past been made between "serious professional misconduct" and incompetence. It rejected the idea that the definition of serious professional misconduct should be widened to include unacceptable or inappropriate conduct of a kind which would not call a doctor's continued registration into question. It also rejected any lowering of the threshold for formal disciplinary proceedings by substituting "professional misconduct" for "serious professional misconduct". Nor did the working party recommend amendment of the 1983 Medical Act along the lines proposed by Nigel Spearing MP to introduce a second, lower tier of "unacceptable professional conduct". NHS issues in the category of "unacceptable conduct" should continue to be dealt with under local NHS disciplinary procedures.

Other recommendations were as follows:

— Initiatives to provide information to patients, both NHS and other, should be taken by local and NHS authorities, Health Councils and consumer and patients' associations. The Council itself should prepare a leaflet about the nature of its own disciplinary jurisdiction and the procedures under which complaints are considered to supplement the individual advice which is already given to complainants.
— No change in the standing instructions whereby NHS patients who complain to the Council are immediately advised by the office to go through NHS procedures in the first instance.[22]
— The GMC should initiate discussions about the improvement of procedures for licensing private clinics, for the appointment of GP locums and for checking the qualifications of doctors employed in the deputising service.
— Lay persons should be involved in the Council's initial screening of disciplinary cases to go forward for committee consideration and matters associated with the formal changes in procedure rules that this would involve.

— Council should convey its view to the Department of Health that lay persons be included in the "intermediate procedures" proposed for the disciplining of NHS hospital consultants (see below, p.124)
— The Department of Health should extend those procedures to junior grades.
— The drafting of charges in conduct cases should be kept under review.

It was also recommended that Council should wait, before making its own proposals, until decisions were made with regard to NHS disciplinary procedures and there had been an opportunity to see how the new procedures were implemented and assessed. These will only apply to NHS hospitals.

The 1989 Annual Report reporting on these developments indicated that amendments to the Medical Act would be needed.[23] According to the *British Medical Journal*,[24] the Council is thinking along the lines of the procedures used to deal with sick doctors. The procedures would be invoked by the GMC when complainants have produced evidence of failure by a doctor to achieve a reasonable standard of performance; this would be followed by assessment by a preliminary screener, in its turn followed by a local performance review. If the local action was unsuccessful the doctor would be referred to a GMC "performance review committee" which would have power to restrict the doctor's registration. After formal consultations the Council aims to bring proposals for approval to the Council in 1991, with a view to legislation in 1992.

The criticisms of the Council's current regulation of the profession, particularly with regard to competence, have come from inside (both medical and lay) and increasingly from outside the Council. The working party clearly had a difficult time attempting to reconcile widely divergent views. It has carefully considered the criticisms, but in a piecemeal manner. In the course of discussion, it will be noted, the concept of "competence" has been changed to one of "performance". The working party did not set out to review the work and role of the GMC in the whole regulatory process of the medical profession. This was not its brief, but according to Lock and Havard that may be what is now needed.[25]

National Health Service

1. Hospital discipline A joint working party of representatives of the Health Departments, the NHS and the professions reviewed the disciplinary procedures for hospital and community doctors and dentists.[26] Their criticisms were directed at the procedures under HM(61)112 which gives guidance to health authorities on disciplinary proceedings against hospital doctors and dentists in matters of professional conduct or competence, particularly where the outcome could involve dismissal, and also at the paragraph 190 procedures for appeal from dismissal.

Among the joint working party's 14 recommendations are ones which intend to ensure that, in all health authorities, disciplinary procedures apply even-handedly to all doctors and dentists and, importantly, to reduce the long drawn out, cumbersome and expensive nature of the existing procedures. The Savage Inquiry,[27] albeit undoubtedly the best publicised, was only one which of recent years had drawn attention to these disadvantages. An important proposal is the suggested establishment of an intermediate procedure, short of the full disciplinary process—sometimes referred to as the ''Three Stern Men''. This would provide that, in cases where there was specific concern about the professional conduct or competence of a consultant or consultants, or where there were major problems arising from differing professional views within a department, the Regional Medical Officer (or his equivalent) could invite the Joint Consultants Committee to nominate assessors to investigate and advise him. Only suggested at present for consultants and not proposed for training grades, the working party suggest that consideration should be given later to the application of such a scheme to associate specialists and other career grades.

2. Complaints procedures Where the joint working party stress the medical review of disciplinary cases, the Association of Community Health Councils for England and Wales (ASCHCEW) stress the importance of lay involvement in complaints procedures. ASCHCEW held a conference in 1988 which reviewed the NHS complaints procedures. They subsequently issued a user's model for a complaints system[28] which was for a year the subject of discussion and comment, after which ASCHCEW issued their considered version of what an appropriate complaints system should look like. Its main provisions are as follows.

— Clear information should be available to the public regarding complaints, including time limits within which complaints should be dealt with.

— All complainants should have access to free, independent and confidential advice on how to complain and to support whilst processing a complaint.

— Whenever a patient, relative or carer is concerned at the standard of health services provided, they should be encouraged to raise the matter immediately with the service provider or officer in charge.

— All complaints should begin with an initial investigation to determine whether conciliation involving discussion and explanation or a full enquiry would be the more appropriate and desirable course of action for the complainant.

— Complainants should have right of access to an "independent complaints investigation service" which, although drawing on the expertise of the health care professions, would be under lay control.

— It should be a condition of contract of all family practitioners, NHS contractors and other health care staff that they shall take part in these procedures as required.

— Complainants should receive a full explanation of the outcome of any enquiries.

— If necessary, the complaint and the results of the investigation should be referred to a Compensation Agency. This would not prejudice the complainant's right of appeal to a Court if the compensation awarded was not satisfactory.

— Where appropriate the complaint and the results of the investigation should be referred to the employing and/or professional body for possible disciplinary action. All parties to the complaint should be informed if such a referral is made, have the right to make an independent complaint and be informed of the outcome of any disciplinary action;

— Any new system should include mechanisms to ensure the accountability of those administering it.[29]

Parliamentary procedures

As an administrative apparatus the NHS is accountable to Parliament through its Board and the Department of Health. In terms of administrative justice the NHS and its staffs are also answerable to the Health Service Commissioner (HSC)—the Ombudsman. The HSC, however, has no jurisdiction over clinical matters; these, in consequence of the still upheld doctrine of clinical autonomy, are subject only to peer review. For junior doctors this means to their consultant in charge, for the fully qualified either to peers in some form of medical audit or to the GMC if allegations of serious professional misconduct are involved. Medical practitioners may be held accountable to the HSC for maladministration in their NHS work, but not for their clinical decisions or actions. In addition, Parliamentary Select Committees (particularly, the Public Accounts and Social Services Select Committees) hold a watching brief on behalf of the state.

Legal

All medical practitioners are subject, as are the rest of us, to the civil and criminal law. The importance of the law with regard to medicine lies in the redress it may be able to offer to aggrieved patients. Patients or their representatives may have recourse to the law in order to establish "the principle of respect for established legal rights or claims of the patient . . . one of which is his (sic) power of determination".[30] Cases may be brought to establish medical accountability to the patient. One reason is to gain compensation for a harm that the patient has suffered. Here the law can only act where negligence has been proved. In this procedure two goals are confused: pecuniary compensation for victims of medical negligence and medical accountability in the interest of that patient and patients at large.

It is doubtful whether the law works well in either regard. The amount of compensation received is a lottery depending on the circumstances of the trial; where negligence is admitted the case is settled privately out of court and little deterrent effect may ensue.[31] In general, there is no guarantee that anything will be done to rectify the situation for the future.[32] Since 1982 increased attention has been drawn to these and other problems by Action for the Victims of Medical Accidents (AVMA).[33] The problems associated with compensation for medical injury and medical accountability have been reviewed by Ham *et al.*[34] They concluded that the shortcomings of the system are as follows:

— the procedures are lengthy and expensive for all concerned;
— only a small proportion of those who suffer medically related injuries get compensation;
— establishing fault and cause in the tort system results in those with similar needs arising from injury being compensated differently;
— there are shortages of appropriately qualified solicitors and of doctors willing to act as expert witnesses;
— the last may not be unconnected with the adversarial nature of the tort system which leads those involved to close ranks;
— any deterrent effect the law might have is weakened by the availability of professional insurance cover and, more recently, Crown indemnity.

Taken together these findings suggest that the law does not work well in providing medical accountability, either to the aggrieved patient or to the public at large, in improving the quality of medical care delivered.

Ham *et al.*[35] also reviewed possible reforms, drawing attention to three options: modifying the existing system and strengthening accountability; introducing a no-fault compensation scheme and providing compensation through social security. Ham *et al.* suggested that in the short term most consideration should be given to proposals to modify the present system viz.:

— providing potential claimants with means of identifying appropriately skilled solicitors;
— increasing publicity for legal services;
— modifying fee-splitting arrangements among lawyers to provide greater incentives to them to pass cases on to colleagues with specialist knowledge and experience;
— making access to legal aid easier;
— making arrangements for pooling risks among health authorities;

— improving and extending medical audits and confidential
enquiries into incidents;
— extending and simplifying disciplinary procedures, both NHS
and GMC;
— establishing the independent investigating panels proposed by
the Davies Committee on Hospital Complaints procedures in
1973 to examine clinical complaints.

These short-term improvements, Ham *et al.* think, would help to
deter doctors from acting negligently and would assist patients
and their relatives to obtain adequate explanations when things
go wrong.

In the longer run, because the adversarial tort system would
still lead to problems about compensation, they also propose a
no-fault compensation system, but learning from the experience
of Sweden and New Zealand by, for example, examining carefully
the accidents to be covered by compensation, ensuring equity
between the treatment of all types of accident victims and the
sick and disabled. Also in the longer term, they suggest
procedures for disciplining doctors on the lines of the Swedish
Medical Responsibility Board, which includes significant lay
participation.[36] Their final proposal is for a single point of
contact for all complaints and guarantees of the genuine
independence of all enquiries into complaints.

No-fault compensation is now BMA policy.[37] It has been the
subject of a Bill in the House of Commons during 1990. It was
discussed by ASCHCEW in 1987,[38] but it is not clear whether
they currently support it since they have proposed the
compensation agency. Reservations arise because no-fault
compensation does not necessarily ensure full investigation of
complaints. For these reasons it is opposed by AVMA.[39]

Accountability in private practice

Those in independent private practice are accountable, as are all
practitioners, to their individual patients for the treatment they
give them and to the General Medical Council for their
professional conduct. Their only other mode of accountability
is through the law. Those employed by a private firm or hospital
are also formally accountable to their employing authority
according to the contracts they have accepted, within the limits

which law, custom and practice may bestow by virtue of their professional membership. Unless serious professional misconduct is involved, in which case a complaint may be made to the GMC, patients in private practice have no procedures available to them except legal ones.

Discussion

Professional self-regulation dominates

This paper has reviewed four types of ways in which members of the medical profession may be called to account, severally or collectively. They were: procedures associated with self-regulation; the NHS, both disciplinary and complaints procedures; Parliamentary procedures, particularly Select Committees and the law. The review has shown how separate each of the four types is from the others, in terms both of intention and execution.

However, the distinctions are less clear cut than one might expect from the intentions of each and the authority under which they are undertaken. The law appears to be the most independent but "the law only ever requires the doctor to act in a way *other reasonable and informed doctors* judge to be proper".[40] According to Professor Kennedy in "all other professions and walks of life, the standard of care by reference to which a person is judged is a matter for the court to determine. Expert evidence is *relevant but not determinative*".[41]

This principle is paramount throughout all the accountability procedures. Not only at law, but in any circumstance in which medical practitioners might be called to account, the profession has insisted that their peers should make the judgments.[42] This insistence has been accepted from the time the modern mode of state involvement in the provision of health care was established. For example, service committees handling complaints in general practice have had lay chairpersons, but the decision-makers are medical. In the GMC itself, although lay persons have been present at disciplinary hearings since 1926,[43] the decision is determined by the medical members, albeit informed by a lay input. Professional self-regulation is clearly implicit in every form of medical accountability. It is the principle of essence. This discussion will therefore focus mainly on self-regulation and particularly on the role of the GMC.

My research conundrum

Professional self-regulation has hazards for the regulators. The most difficult conundrum which I have tried to unravel has been as follows. The Council's members and leaders are people of high ethical standards who care about the delivery of a good health service, believe they are doing a good job and continually strive to do better. Yet they operate and support a system of regulation which neither ensures the continuing competence of practitioners, nor adequately disciplines the incompetent. Nor is the system really sensitive or accessible to the members of the public they seek to serve—it is almost as if the public had become the enemy to be kept at bay. Furthermore, and here is the serious difficulty, most (but not all) medical members of the GMC *really do not understand* the size of the gap between what it is supposed to do (judged by statements in Merrison and the instructions in the Act) and what the Council actually does.

Differing perspectives of profession and patient

Unconditional self-regulation is not accepted by everybody as providing appropriate safeguards. ASCHCEW, with experience of guarding the public interest so far as the health service is concerned, are not in favour of this principle. Their proposal, noted above, was for an independent complaints investigation service with medical advice but under lay control. As things stand such a proposal (quite apart from what might be government's view of its financial implications) is unlikely to be acceptable to the medical profession. But would it be so seriously against the profession's interests? Could it even be in the professional interest?

At one level it is probably true that the best interests of the patient are also the best interest of the profession. However, in matters of accountability, the different perspectives of patient and public compared with profession and practitioner tend to be stressed. The distinction is sometimes put in terms of the public being concerned with outcome while the profession is concerned with process. That the profession itself should monitor outcome in medical audits is increasingly widely accepted, as has been shown above. But the GMC's Working Party Report felt that a major problem exists because small "lapses" on the part of the practitioner may lead to a more serious outcome for the patient than might a serious error.[44] This reiterates the classical medical focus on process, or the general level of performance, rather than on outcome.

Reassessment of professional self-regulation needed

The sort of questions which have to be addressed are: What is professional self-regulation for? In whose interest does it, or could it, work? What are its advantages and disadvantages and from whose point of view? In the profession's own interest questions such as these should be thoroughly aired. The profession was probably misguided to have prevented the Merrison Committee on the regulation of the profession[45] from discussing the principle. The political climate then was far less hostile to the professions than it is now.[46] However, that is past history and the issue can no longer be ducked.

1. The changes already made   The GMC can justly claim that it has changed a great deal in the last 10 years. The mode of dealing with sick doctors is generally agreed to be a great advance on the situation before the 1978 Medical Act. The proportion, as well as the number, of lay members has been increased during the 1980s. A lay person is now involved in initial disciplinary screening; for some time there has even been a lay person on the Finance Committee; there are now two lay members on disciplinary hearings, not just one as formerly. Furthermore, it was the GMC, not the joint working party, which suggested the introduction of lay persons into the proposed intermediate disciplinary procedures. Council may not approve of proposals for lay control,[47] but they have taken the lesson about the importance of a lay presence.

Council's ethical guidelines (the blue pamphlet) have made it much plainer that bad practice as well as bad behaviour may constitute serious professional misconduct.[48] In the past 10 years more cases involving clinical practice have been passed through to the Professional Conduct Committee, but seem still to be dealt with more leniently than other conduct offences.[49] "There but for the grace of God . . ." tempers judgments. It has been my belief that really bad practice could always have been construed as serious professional misconduct (and indeed was in gross cases). That more cases were not brought forward was more a matter of will on the part of the members than the powers of the GMC. There is now no doubt about their powers since the judgment about a dentist.[50] Council is in a position to join those who are setting the tone for the profession that self-regulation does include monitoring outcome. Routinely to treat serious clinical errors as serious professional misconduct would constitute a major change in the way professional self-regulation has hitherto been understood, as would setting up any competence procedures under the heading of professional self-regulation.

2. Changes yet to come   Council accepted the report of the working party on disciplinary procedure in May 1989. As noted above, procedures modelled on the GMC's Health Committee (used to handle complaints against sick doctors) are being developed with the intention of assessing the performance of doctors against whom allegations of incompetence have been made. The Council hopes the proposals will be agreed by the profession and Council in 1991 for legislation in 1992.

Many struggles and difficulties have already been experienced in getting agreement this far; no doubt others are yet to come. It seems likely that in looking at performance, rather than outcome or competence in any one incident, the Council may have found a formula upon which doctors' leaders can agree. From the professional perspective the GMC has moved a great deal. From the lay point of view, until details are known, the suggested local aspects of the procedures raise doubts as to how fair and open they may be.

There is still a long road to travel if professional regulation is to catch up with the conditions of late 20th century medicine, of the modern state and the market place. In this light the changes the GMC has made seem less impressive. The details of the performance procedures are not yet to hand. The working party report, after two years of hard work, was disappointing in that it appeared defensive, dealing piecemeal with particular criticisms, recommending the Council wait for others before it acted, passing as much as possible to other authorities and making no strong proposals about how to deal with problems which arise in private medicine.[51] It now seems possible that the performance formula may be a way of, yet again, ducking outcome. Let us hope not. But why the slowness and the timidity?

Origins of self-regulation: unity, service, exclusiveness

The power and character of the medical profession owe much to its unity, the high value it places on service, and its exclusiveness. The last especially is also a source of its present problems and impedes vision about solutions.

Historically the *unity* of the profession, based on the principle that all the medically qualified are equals, has been a source of professional strength and independence. The unity, the strong sense of shared membership and the institutions which sustain it (among which the GMC is important), have played a part in enhancing the quality of medical practice and the status of the profession. In the present turmoil associated with the NHS Review,[52] the National Health Service and Community Care Act 1990 and the challenges to the profession,[53] its unity may be threatened, as it was in 1968.

The concept of *service*, central to the concept of profession, still motivates medical practitioners. The profession has provided the public, not only with—on the whole—excellent medical practitioners, but also with a body whose representatives can speak with a strong voice to governments and other powerful institutions on behalf of the public health, curative and preventative. This citizen would not wish to lose such a champion, especially in these days of increased centralisation of government, large-scale industrial production and nuclear hazard.

The *exclusiveness* of the profession, which derives from the unique and common training experienced by all medical practitioners, has three effects. First, it leads to the isolation of the profession with its characteristic in-turningness and seeming arrogance. Second, it creates a gap between practitioner and patient—a gap which is not well understood in the profession, being seen as a problem in the mode of communication, whereas much of the problem derives from differing experiential and knowledge bases. Third, the exclusiveness creates for its members a faith in the value to them as individuals of the institutional arrangements established—a kind of "subjective illusion".[54] In the early days of the establishment of the profession the exclusiveness was used to establish the profession over against the many other types of practitioners that still abounded then. Controlling themselves, controlling their education, restraining the excesses of their brethren (no women practitioners in those days) were all among the ways in which 19th century medical practitioners succeeded in convincing patients to call upon them, rather than other kinds of healers, and finally convinced the state to support them above all others.

The exclusiveness brought power. Since the 1858 Medical Act, successive governments have consulted registered medical practitioners with regard to health matters. All appointments of practitioners made by government and its agents are drawn from among the registered. Consequently in all authorities at all levels, medical doctors are in post and able to influence events if not control them—and are present, furthermore, in greater numbers and with better remuneration than any other single category of health care workers. To all observers, whatever may be doctors' own uncertainties, medicine appears powerful and privileged.

Perhaps it is collective memory of the early struggle to exclude the unqualified from practice which has led medical practitioners ever since to be constantly uncertain of their security, and to feel beleaguered and vulnerable.[55] They probably have more reason for these feelings now than ever before. What the professions collectively, and medicine among them, have apparently not yet understood is that they have to a considerable extent brought the present attack upon themselves.[56] Watkins[57] argues that it has been this exclusiveness, the refusal to share power—with patients' groups, other professions, other health workers—which has led medicine to be cast in the role of an "oppressor". If this is not understood by the profession the danger in the present situation is that defensive professional strategies will reinforce the hostility and risk losing popular support.

Hazards of self-regulation for the profession
My conundrum of how well-meaning and well-intentioned people could apparently deceive themselves about the nature of

what they were doing can partly be explained by this exclusiveness. It can also partly be explained by the inevitable consequences of control in a hierarchical mode. Together these processes amount to hazards for the professions which lurk in professional self-regulation.

As Professor Dorothy Smith[58], writing in another context but relevant to our concerns, has pointed out, people who are involved in the work of ruling (or regulating) come to view the world in distinctive ways. They share problems, experiences, concerns and interests in their committees and councils with others similarly placed.[59] These experiences of the regulators are particular to them and markedly different from those of the people they are controlling—albeit they are also medical practitioners. The continual focus on these everyday problems of governing can lead a ruling elite to become out of touch with its own rank and file as well as with those it seeks to serve. Yet the elite's authority and power depends upon the silences of those who do not participate, who are outside the process. When the silences are broken wise rulers meet their critics openly: I believe the GMC's troubles of 1968 and thereafter were compounded by secretiveness and defensive intransigence. The profession has no space in the 1990s to risk the disunity of a rift between medical leaders and front line practitioners.

This is not a conspiracy theory of medicine against the laity or of medical leaders against the rank and file of doctors. I am suggesting that the regulation of the profession might work better, one hazard might be removed, if regulatory procedures were more open, and involved a wider range of medical practitioners, a wider range of health workers and a wider range of persons who can represent patients and the public, and if there were much more and freer dialogue among all these categories at every level of the service. The improved public relations which the GMC has recently established[60] acknowledge this need, but go only a small way towards meeting it.

The specialness of medicine

The unique nature of medical work has been a main justification for its special position at law and in disciplinary matters. Medicine is indeed special: as well as dealing with matters of life and death, the nature of its relationships with its clients is distinctive. No doctor can practise medicine satisfactorily without the cooperation of the patient whose body and/or mind s/he is working on. The patient's input is essential to any treatment and contributes to the outcome. Patients are better looked upon as partners in the treatment process than as consumers of a market product.[61] As active participants in their own care patients have interests in the competence assurance procedures relating to the practitioners who serve them and in any disciplinary actions that may take place. To shut them out as much as has hitherto been done will continue to raise the hostility the profession so much fears. To continue in the old mode could be more dangerous for the profession at this time than sharing its power.

The way forward

There are two facets to finding solutions to our present dilemmas. One has to do with the principles which should guide medical regulation as we move into the 21st century. In this context the questions identified earlier are relevant: What is professional self-regulation for? In whose interest does it, or could it, work? What are its advantages and disadvantages and from whose point of view?

In terms of the underlying principle the answer seems to be that regulation, whosoever does it, should be (i) in the interests of the profession such that its members shall be deemed trustworthy, and (ii) in the interests of patients and potential patients such that they may know where they can place their trust. Ensuring continuing high standards of practice and conduct is necessary to both professionals and patients. Present arrangements under all the four types of accountability discussed in this paper do not ensure this.

The second facet of the solution-finding exercise is to discover improved ways of achieving the ends of good regulation. This involves improvements in the accountability arrangements themselves.

1. Redefining profession The first task is to redefine the concept of profession and its regulation in the light of the contemporary medical, social and political realities, to retain

what is of value—the concept of service, for example—and to
shed the out-of-date. Much modern health care is not based on
a one-to-one relationship. It is a team effort. The concept of
"health profession" needs to take account of this. Ideally, it
should also be recognised and reflected in all accountability
procedures. Patients also, as I have argued, are part of the health
care team.

2. Open discussions As a first step in this process of
redefinition I would invite the profession in these troubled times
to find ways of meeting the rest of us in the search for solutions
to our mutual problems. The profession can afford to do this on
a basis of equality thereby retaining and reinforcing its valuable
sense of service and enhancing the true sense of profession. What
is needed is genuine discussions, not exchanges of postures.

3. Revised procedures So far as the second facet is
concerned, I would not wish to be prescriptive at this stage as
to the structures which might be proposed by such a collective
investigation, for I would wish to hear the views of all
participants before coming to detailed conclusions. However, in
the preceding discussion I have indicated some improvements in
practice which I think it is urgent to consider. So far as these are
concerned there is an ideal position which one might like to
work towards and certain immediate steps which could be taken
to ameliorate some of the present difficulties.

*4. Procedures acceptable to practitioners—and to
patients* To start with it is important to note that any system
of regulation works better if those involved recognise the need
for it, take part in its establishment, agree that the system is fair
and legitimate and trust the way it is operated. In the case of
medicine this is relevant for both disciplinary and complaints
procedures.

Medical audit is one important contribution to this end, which
practitioners themselves are installing. I am delighted with the
intention that medical audit should become universal. Let us
hope obstacles to its extension can be overcome without delay.
For myself I shall be more delighted when the profession feels

strong enough to include other health care professionals and patients in many aspects of their audit process. As it is, medicine itself is insufficiently united in the audit process. There is not yet one system on which all medical specialisms agree and join together in promulgating. NCEPOD has gone further than previous attempts at self-assessment of performance and outcome in having many major Colleges and Faculties involved.

5. Compensation for medical accidents The BMA supports no-fault compensation[62] while making it clear this should not be used as a way of evading the consequences of negligence.[63] Undoubtedly our present court procedures do not serve either the profession or the public well. Havard[64] discusses investigative procedures which would ensure that any negligence, incompetence or accident is uncovered and, so far as possible, prevented for the future. I would be pleased if the BMA were to argue for thorough procedures of that kind, but allied with a system of universal taxation-based compensation for those who need it, whatever the cause of their injury or disability. This seems likely to be the most economical as well as equitable way to handle misfortune in a civilised society, preferable both to no-fault and to the present system, which, as we have seen, has all the characteristics of a lottery.

6. An integrated set of accountability procedures Some way certainly has to be found whereby, when something has gone wrong, doctors are not subjected to multiple and repetitive enquiries: this is too oppressive, and sometimes leads the GMC to be soft when it should be tough on a doctor who is before it after other disciplinary appearances. One integrated set of accountability procedures is surely enough for patients as well as doctors. The law apart, the multiplicity of systems is itself a commentary on failures of self-regulation. Had that worked really satisfactorily, government would not have found it necessary to bring in so many other procedures, from hospitals complaints to the control of dangerous drugs. The problem presented by the small lapse on the part of a generally competent and conscientious doctor which eventuates in serious consequences for the patient would not loom so large as it does to the GMC if there were good regulatory procedures throughout the profession, such as medical audit could provide. Accountability for the proper expenditure of public funds will always be necessary in medicine as elsewhere.

7. *A single point of entry*   Until we have an integrated system combining complaints, discipline and accountability procedures, however, members of the public do need to have, as of right, a single point of entry into the grievance system where they can get advice as to which way they should proceed. Such a point should be provided in localities throughout the country, perhaps by enhanced Community Health Councils.

8. *A totally new kind of GMC?*   A unified system would have to cover private as well as NHS health care. It would also imply the disappearance of the GMC as we know it today. The mode of enquiry into medical mishaps in Sweden described by Professor Marilynn Rosenthal[65] has much to commend it, representing better the realities of modern health care than does our fragmentary and hierarchical system. In Sweden all health care professionals and lay persons are involved. But doctors may be comforted: theirs remains the strongest voice.

In the meantime, while such a system is being worked out, further changes to the GMC are needed. I would suggest that other health care professionals should sit on the GMC as of right—initially after the 1978 Act a nurse was appointed, and there has always been one since; now a pharmacist is also an appointed member, but all go under the guise of lay people. There should be a great many more representatives of patients and potential patients. In the run up to the 1978 Medical Act radical doctors successfully argued that the proportion of GMC members elected by the body of registered medical practitioners should constitute a majority over nominated and appointed members together. The case for public representatives, the "truly lay" having an overall majority is probably stronger than was the case of the medical electorate.

9. *Time to shed the illusions*   These may seem frighteningly radical proposals, but I believe the time has come for the

profession to shed long-cherished illusions. Sir Raymond Hoffenberg argued in the 1986 Rock Carling Lecture that clinical freedom is "of course, a chimera": personal, moral, ethical and even legal constraints on clinical decisions have always existed and been observed.[66] Hoffenberg further argues that the medical profession is mistaken in continuing to believe in this chimera as a guide to their actions.[67] His recognition of the illusory nature of clinical freedom is encouraging. That belief is part of the collective "subjective illusion", which I mentioned earlier, and which the profession has clung to over the years.

There are similar chimeric qualities in other aspects of professional self-regulation. The ancient structures which the profession so anxiously defends are not so relevant as once they were, nor any longer so personally useful to members. The profession would do well to take them apart and throw away the illusory aspects. There is, for example, no need to cling to the special expert status whereby only doctors can determine what is right in medical matters. My experience suggests that, given medical advice, non-medical persons are perfectly able to come to wise conclusions.

Any group of workers—and here medicine is no exception—is right to keep as much control over the working lives of its members as it can. I have no desire to see the profession dismantled in that sense. In the public interest I trust medical practitioners remain strong and united. However, none of us can escape the requirement to be accountable.

I for one am looking to the profession for a vigorous lead towards a better mode of regulation—one which does not duck the outcome issue and which does not constantly wait for others to move first. The GMC is uniquely placed to give the lead by transforming itself and thus helping in the wider transformation that is necessary.

Acknowledgements

A grant from the ESRC, GOO 232247, made possible the research on the General Medical Council. This is gratefully acknowledged, as is the help and cooperation from two past Presidents and the present President of the Council, the past and present Registrars, and many members who agreed to be interviewed or who corresponded with me. Thanks also to all those others who helped by being interviewed about the GMC; to the librarians of Warwick University, the Barnes Library, the Royal Society of Medicine; to the Royal College of Physicians of London and the Royal College of Surgeons of England, ASCHCEW, AVMA and the King's Fund for providing information; and thanks to Judy Morris for help with data collection and analysis as well as with secretarial work. For the last, thanks also to Eileen Clark. Part of the analysis and writing up was done while I held the Lucile Petry Leone Professorship in the Department of Social and Behavioral Sciences of the School of Nursing, University of California, San Francisco: my thanks to them. Professor Margot Jefferys read and commented on an earlier draft. My thanks to her and also to Mr J. Lunn and Mr B. Devlin for their help. Wiley Medical have agreed to publish a book on the GMC based on the research. Finally, thanks to all those who helped in other ways, especially Jennifer Lorch for her support.

Notes and references

1. This paper was first presented to a meeting arranged by the King's Fund Institute and the Centre for Medical Law and Ethics of King's College on 30 November 1989. I am grateful to them for setting the meeting up. Its purpose conformed very much with what I believe to be urgently necessary. So far as any proposed changes in medical accountability are concerned, my view has been that "from the start, doctors, patients, and potential patients [should] work openly together to improve the system" (M. Stacey, "A sociologist looks at the GMC" (1989) *Lancet* 713). In the paper I shall discuss only the accountability of registered medical practitioners. There are important questions about the accountability of practitioners who work in a variety of healing modalities other than those registered by the General Medical Council. *Au fond* the principles which should govern their accountability are essentially the same as for those presently registered by the Council. However, for historical reasons their circumstances are in many ways different and cannot be dealt with here.

2. P. Day and R. Klein, *Accountabilities: Five Public Services* (London and New York: Tavistock, 1987).

3. See, for example, M. S. Larson, *The Rise of Professionalism* (Berkeley, California: University of California Press, 1977); I. Waddington, *The Medical Profession in the Industrial Revolution* (Dublin: Gill and Macmillan, 1984).

4. *Report of the Committee of Inquiry into the Regulation of the Medical Profession* [Merrison], (London: HMSO, 1975) p.3.

5. *Report of the Committee on Hospital Complaints Procedure* [Davies], (London: HMSO, 1973).

6. H. B. Devlin, "Professional audit: quality control; keeping up to date", in *Some Aspects of Anaesthetic Safety: Clinical Anaesthesiology* (vol. 2, no. 2, London: Baillière Tindall, 1988) pp. 299–324; H. B. Devlin, "Audit and the quality of clinical care", (1990) 72 *Supplement to the Annals of the Royal College of Surgeons of England* (no. 1) 3–14; C. D. Shaw, "Acceptability of audit", (1980) 281 *British Medical Journal* 1443–5.
7. N. Buck, H. B. Devlin and I. N. Lunn, *The Report of a Confidential Enquiry into Perioperative Deaths* (London: Nuffield Provincial Hospitals Trust and King's Fund, London, 1987); J. N. Lunn and H. B. Devlin, "Lessons from the Confidential Enquiry into Perioperative Deaths in three NHS Regions" (1987) *Lancet* 1384–6.
8. H. B. Devlin, "Audit and the quality of clinical care" (1990) 72 *Supplement to the Annals of the Royal College of Surgeons of England* (no. 1) 3–14.
9. See the review of C. M. McKee, M. Lauglo and L. Lessof, "Medical audit: a review" (1989) 82 *Journal of the Royal Society of Medicine* 474–8, but note also M. D. Vickers, "Medical Audit" (1989) 82 *Journal of the Royal Society of Medicine* 773.
10. J. Wilmot, "Review of medical audit" (1990) 83 *Journal of the Royal Society of Medicine* 58–9.
11. *What Sort of Doctor? Report from General Practice 23* (London: Royal College of General Practitioners, 1985).
12. *Working for Patients* (London: HMSO, 1989).
13. *Medical Audit: a First Report: What, Why and How?* (London: The Royal College of Physicians of London, 1989); *Guidelines to Clinical Audit in Surgical Practice* (London: The Royal College of Surgeons of England, 1989).
14. C. M. McKee, M. Lauglo and L. Lessof, supra note 9, p. 474.
15. W. van't Hoff, "Welcome to medical audit" (1989) 298 *British Medical Journal* 1021–3; C. M. McKee, M. Lauglo and L. Lessof, supra note 9.
16. J. Walton, "The General Medical Council: past, present and future", *The Lord Cohen History of Medicine Lecture,* mimeo.
17. *Report of the Committee of Inquiry into the Regulation of the Medical Profession* [Merrison], (London: HMSO, 1975), p. 3.
18. Ibid.
19. I. Kennedy, *The Unmasking of Medicine* (London: Granada, 1983) p. 177; R. Klein and A. Shinebourne, "Doctors' discipline" (1972) 22 *New Society* p. 399–401; J. Robinson, *A Patient Voice at the GMC: a Lay Member's View of the General Medical Council* (London: Health Rights Report 1, 1988) esp. pp. 33–4; M. Stacey, "A sociologist looks at the GMC" (1989) *Lancet* (April 1st) 714; M. Stacey, "The British General Medical Council and medical ethics", in G. Weisz, ed. *Social Science Perspectives on Medical Ethics* (Dordrecht: Kluwer Academic, 1990) pp. 163–84.
20. *Report of the Working Party on the Council's Disciplinary Procedures in Response to Allegations of Failure to Provide a Good*

Standard of Medical Care (London: General Medical Council, press notice, 25/5/89).

21. "Report of the Working Party on the Council's Disciplinary Procedures in Response to Allegations of Failure to Provide a Good Standard of Medical Care" (London: General Medical Council, mimeo 25/4/89).

22. A matter strongly criticised by Jean Robinson, *A Patient Voice at the GMC: a lay member's view of the General Medical Council* (London: Health Rights Report, 1988).

23. *Annual Report, 1989* (London: General Medical Council, 1989) pp. 2, 7.

24. "GMC moving on competence" (1990) 301 *British Medical Journal* 1116.

25. S. Lock, "Regulating doctors: a good case for the profession to set up a new enquiry" (1989) 299 *British Medical Journal* 137-8; J. D. J. Havard, *Medical Negligence: the Mounting Dilemma,* The Stevens Lecture for the Laity (London: Royal Society of Medicine, 1989).

26. *Disciplinary Procedures for Hospital and Community Doctors and Dentists: Report of the Joint Working Party* (London: Crown Copyright, August, 1989).

27. W. Savage, *A Savage Enquiry* (London: Virago, 1986); W. Savage, P. Bousquet, G. Cardy, P. Tomlin, "Disciplining doctors" (1988) 296 *British Medical Journal* 1674; W. Savage, "Disciplining hospital consultants" (1989) 289 *British Medical Journal* 1404; I. Kennedy, "Review of the year 2: Confidentiality, competence and malpractice", in P. Byrne, *Medicine in Contemporary Society: King's College Studies 1986-7* (London: King Edward's Hospital Fund for London, 1987) pp. 49-63.

28. *NHS Complaints Procedures: a Report of a Conference Held 11/10/88,* Health News Briefing (London: Association of Community Health Councils for England and Wales, 1989).

29. *NHS Complaints Procedures: a Review by the Association of Community Health Councils for England and Wales* (London: Association of Community Health Councils for England and Wales, 1990).

30. I. Kennedy, *The Unmasking of Medicine* (London: Granada, 1983) p. 172.

31. Ibid. pp. 173-8; C. Ham, R. Dingwall, P. Fenn and D. Harris, *Medical Negligence: Compensation and Accountability* (London: King's Fund Institute, 1988) p. 26.

32. A. Simanowitz, "Medical accidents: the problem and the challenge", in P. Byrne, *Medicine in Contemporary Society: King's College Studies 1986-7* (London: King Edward's Hospital Fund for London, 1987) p. 118.

33. Simanowitz, ibid.; *Annual Report, 1989* (London: Action for Victims of Medical Accidents, 1989) pp. 4-5.

34. C. Ham, R. Dingwall, P. Fenn and D. Harris, *Medical Negligence: Compensation and Accountability* (London: King's Fund Institute, 1988).

35. Ibid.

36. M. M. Rosenthal, *Dealing with Medical Malpractice: the British and Swedish Experience* (London: Tavistock, 1987).

37. Report of the No Fault Compensation Working Party (London: British Medical Association, 1987).

38. "When Things Go Wrong in the NHS: Compensation and Investigation, 1987", in *NHS Complaints Procedures: a Review by the Association of Community Health Councils for England and Wales* (London: Association of Community Health Councils for England and Wales, 1990) app. iv.

39. *Compensation for Medical Injury Bill* (London: Action for Victims of Medical Accidents, mimeo, AJS/HKLM, 26/10/90, 1990); A. Simanowitz, paper read to RSM/BSA meeting 12/13 January 1988 at the Royal College of Physicians.

40. I. Kennedy, "Review of the year 2: Confidentiality, competence and malpractice" in P. Byrne, *Medicine in Contemporary Society: King's College Studies 1986–7* (London: King Edward's Hospital Fund for London, 1987) p. 59, his emphasis.

41. Ibid. p. 59, my emphasis; but see J. D. J. Havard, *Medical Negligence: the Mounting Dilemma,* The Stevens Lecture for the Laity (London: Royal Society of Medicine, 1989), pp. 12–13 on expert disagreements.

42. A good example may be found in the "Grey Book", the bible of the 1974 reorganization, *Management Arrangements for the Reorganized National Health Service* (London: DHSS, 1972) 1.18 as follows:

"The management arrangements required for the NHS are different from those commonly used in other large organizations because the work is different. The distinguishing characteristic of the NHS is that to do their work properly, consultants and general practitioners must have clinical autonomy, so that they can be fully responsible for the treatment they prescribe for their patients. It follows that these doctors and dentists work as each other's equals and that they are their own managers. In ethics and in law they are accountable to their patients for the care they prescribe, and they cannot be held accountable to the NHS authorities for the quality of their clinical judgements so long as they act within the broad limits of acceptable medical practice and within policy for the use of resources."

43. W. Pyke-Lees, *Centenary of the General Medical Council* (London: General Medical Council, 1958).

44. The GMC working party (1989) while agreeing that profession and public have shared interests in reducing incompetence (para A3) says at para A2:

"In approaching its task the Working Party accepted that the divergent expectations of the public and profession in relation to the functioning of the Council's disciplinary procedures cannot be completely reconciled. For example, where there is public criticism of a decision of the Professional Conduct Committee, this often arises because of the different perceptions of patients and doctors as to what constitutes serious professional misconduct. In particular, many patients not unnaturally tend to expect the sanctions against a doctor to reflect the seriousness of the consequences of any neglect of professional responsibilities rather than the magnitude of the lapse. A relatively minor failure may have severe consequences for a patient, whereas a far more heinous lapse can have only trivial consequences."

45. *Report of the Committee of Inquiry into the Regulation of the Medical Profession,* (London: HMSO, 1975).
46. M. Stacey, "The General Medical Council and Professional Accountability" (1989) 4 *Public Policy and Administration* (no. 1) 12–27.
47. For example, D. Green, *Which doctor? A Critical Analysis of Professional Barriers to Competition in Health Care* (London: Institute of Economic Affairs, 1985).
48. J. Walton, supra note 16; M. Stacey, "The British General Medical Council and medical ethics", in G. Weisz, ed., *Social Science Perspectives on Medical Ethics* (Dordrecht: Kluwer Academic, 1990) pp. 163–84.
49. R. Smith, "Profile of the GMC: Discipline II: the preliminary screener—a powerful gatekeeper" (1989) 298 *British Medical Journal* 1569–71; R. Smith, "Profile of the GMC: Discipline III: the final stages" (1989) 298 *British Medical Journal* 1632–4; M. Stacey, "The British General Medical Council and medical ethics", in G. Weisz, ed., *Social Science Perspectives on Medical Ethics* (Dordrecht: Kluwer Academic, 1990) pp. 163–84.
50. *Doughty* v. *General Dental Council.*
51. See, for example, D. Campbell, "An investigative journalist looks at medical ethics" (1989) 298 *British Medical Journal* 1171–2; R. Smith "Doctors, unethical treatments and turning a blind eye" (1989) 298 *British Medical Journal* 498–9; S. Lock, "Regulating doctors: a good case for the profession to set up a new enquiry" (1989) 299 *British Medical Journal* 137–8, on the Sharp and Sultan affair, and J. Robinson, *A Patient Voice at the GMC: a Lay Member's View of the General Medical Council* (London: Health Rights Report 1, 1988) p. 20.
52. *Working for Patients* (London: HMSO, 1989).
53. *Review of Restrictive Trade Practices Policy: a Consultative Document,* DTI. (London: HMSO, 1988); questions from the Monopolies and Mergers Commission in 1988 to the professions resulted in the relaxation of restrictions on advertising: see *Services of Medical Practitioners* (London: HMSO, 1989) Cm 582.
54. M. S. Larson, *The Rise of Professionalism* (Berkeley, California: University of California Press, 1977).
55. S. Watkins, *Medicine and Labour: the Politics of a Profession* (London: Lawrence and Wishart, 1988) pp. 117–19.
56. Ibid. p. 18.
57. Ibid.

58. D. Smith, *The Everyday World as Problematic* (Milton Keynes: The Open University Press) pp. 56-7.
59. Richard Smith, for example, has commented on how large the GMC's internal problems loom to its staff and members. R. Smith, "Profile of the GMC: the Council's internal problems" (1989) 299 *British Medical Journal* 40-3.
60. *Annual Report 1989* (London: GMC, 1989) p. 2.
61. M. Stacey, "The health service consumer: a sociological misconception?" in M. Stacey, ed., *The Sociology of the National Health Service*, Sociological Review Monograph 22 (Keele: The University of Keele, 1976).
62. *Report of the No Fault Compensation Working Party* (London: British Medical Association, 1987).
63. See also J. D. J. Havard, *Medical Negligence: the Mounting Dilemma*, The Stevens Lecture for the Laity (London: Royal Society of Medicine, 1989) pp. 17-18.
64. Ibid. pp. 24-6.
65. M. M. Rosenthal, *Dealing with Medical Malpractice: the British and Swedish Experience* (London: Tavistock, 1987).
66. R. Hoffenberg, *Clinical Freedom,* The Rock Carling Fellowship, 1986 (London: The Nuffield Provincial Hospitals Trust, 1987) p. ix.
67. See, for example, his discussion of the reaction to the limited drugs list, ibid. p. 29.

Does the National Health Service have a purpose?

David Seedhouse

This paper makes out the basic case for a philosophical review of the National Health Service. A philosophical review would differ from the conventional health service review by focusing in the first instance upon questions of *purpose*—what is the basic rationale of the health service? what is the health service essentially for?—rather than questions of *process*—how can existing services be delivered more effectively? how might the NHS perform its functions at less financial cost?[1] The paper contends that traditional NHS reviews have chosen the wrong point of departure. Each review has focused on a particular aspect of the operation of the health service. Each has assessed the procedures of the organisation, but not its purpose.

There is a widely held assumption that there is general consensus about the purpose of the NHS. But this supposition is seriously mistaken. Some people share some beliefs about the goals of the NHS but there are many incompatible views of purpose abroad in the organisation. In addition, NHS staff and members of the public often have quite different perceptions of health service objectives. For example, doctors are habitually concerned with medical service costs and government regulations while many lay people believe, perhaps naively, that health care is meant to improve the human condition.[2] These conflicting visions of purpose hinder rational planning, can provoke dispute amongst the various sections of the service, and can cause tension between health workers and their patients.

The fundamental aim of each NHS review has been to make things run more smoothly (and more cheaply). However, because many of the factors which disrupt the efficient functioning of the health service stem from the existence of disparate visions of NHS purpose (the rivalry between the nursing and medical professions is one example) no amount of *process engineering* will produce harmony. What is needed is clarification of the sundry perceptions of purpose, careful analysis of these alternatives, and then open debate about health service purpose until a satisfactory conclusion is reached. This paper is a short and tentative first step towards this goal.

Traditions untouched by reviews

Health services in Britain are reviewed periodically. Each review is initiated in the belief that one or more functions of the existing service ought to be improved. For example, past reviews have focused on improving administration,[3] management structure,[4] and on creating internal markets.[5] Each new review makes recommendations which have massive implications for the people most directly concerned with their implementation, but each time many aspects of the health service are unaltered. Whatever the administrative hierarchy, whoever manages, and whether or not health care finances are directly controlled by government, a massive residue of traditions and expectations persist untouched by conventional health service reviews.

Many traditions have persisted from before the inauguration of the NHS up to the present day. For example, whatever the emphasis of reviews clinicians have remained in especially powerful positions within the health service; resources continue to be allocated according to political muscle rather than generally agreed schemes; pharmaceutical companies persist with persuasive and costly promotions of their products to doctors; "alternative" or "complementary" therapies such as osteopathy and acupuncture endure only as officially unsanctioned last resorts; patients still experience lengthy waits for non-emergency treatment; and "medical education" continues to be little more than repetitive training in clinical knowledge and method. But traditions such as these are not sacrosanct and ought also to be systematically and simultaneously reviewed. This, however, is no simple matter. Currently four factors stand in the way of such a comprehensive review.

Four obstacles to a comprehensive health service review

1. The NHS is extraordinarily large and complex

The provision of health services is currently so broad and diverse that any realistic review of function will be able to concentrate only on certain features of the NHS. It is impossible for even the largest "working party" to understand simultaneously all the processes (and combinations of process) of the NHS.

2. Partly as a result of this complexity the NHS does not possess an overall plan, and in this sense is not a rational organisation

Even if every planned process of the NHS could be comprehended by a study group this would still not be sufficient to understand the organisation fully. Much of what happens in the health service simply *emerges* as the unintended consequence of many disparate plans and processes. One of the largest civilian organisations in the world has, to a significant degree, a life of its own. In 1972, after an extensive study of the NHS, a Minister of Health wrote:

> For the imbalances and the gaps Governments must take their share of the responsibility. Resources were and still are stretched. The acute services had a legitimate priority. *But the shortcomings were not rational. They did not result from a calculation as to the best way to deploy scarce resources. They just happened.*[6] (my italics)

3. There are numerous vested interests within the NHS, many of which have substantial power to lobby for their point of view, and to resist any changes which might be recommended

A huge structure of laws, regulations and mutually beneficial relationships ensures that, short of war or startlingly radical Parliamentary legislation, wholescale reform of the working arrangements of the NHS is virtually inconceivable.

4. A vital distinction between the process and the purpose of health services has consistently been overlooked

All working organisations have both purpose(s) and process(es), both of which can be assessed and both of which might be changed through deliberate policy. Previous reviews have analysed *process* exclusively while simply assuming: (a) the existence of consensus about the purpose of health services, and (b) that this supposed consensus is the only desirable purpose (or set of purposes) for a health service.

All health service reviews so far (including the 1944 White Paper) have taken it as read that the *purpose* of health care is clear, known and agreed. But this is not the case. Analysis shows that there is a range of different conceptions of the nature of health care. Significant, although often covert, disagreement exists within and between the various health service professions, and between the professions and the users of health services.

There is little that any review can do about obstacle 1, short of disbanding the NHS. And without a review of purpose there is little that can be done about obstacles 2 and 3. However, since part of the reason for the lack of an overall plan for the NHS, and part of the reason why vested interests are able to fight their own corners so effectively, is the fact that the purpose of the health service is not clear, a review of purpose could have a liberating effect on future reformers. The path towards a comprehensive review of the NHS can begin only through a philosophical investigation into purpose.

Demonstrating the lack of consensus

In order for a petition for a philosophical review of health services to have credibility it is necessary to establish beyond doubt that there is no consensus over health service purpose. This can be achieved by stressing three points.

1. Unlike a commercial organisation the NHS does not have an obviously supreme purpose

It has been asserted recently that it is quite legitimate to think of the NHS as a business.[7] If this were true then it ought to be possible to regard the health service as analogous to a supermarket chain. But this comparison will not stand up to serious scrutiny. This can be illustrated by reference to a reported conversation between a health service manager and Roy Griffiths, the managing director of Sainsbury—a person charged with a previous conventional review of NHS process.

I went to see Roy Griffiths in his office at Sainsbury's (sic) and while I was talking to him, his secretary handed him a piece of paper. He looked at it and said, "OK". I asked him, "What do you mean 'OK'?" and he said, "My organisation is OK today." It turned out he had just six measures on that piece of paper and from those he could tell what the state of Sainsbury's health had been the day before; things like the amount of money taken yesterday, the freshness quotient—the amount of stuff still on the shelves, the proportion of staff on duty, and so on.[8]

Naturally an efficient organisation such as Sainsbury ought to be able to distill its measures of success or failure into simple categories which make sense to any member of the company. Naturally, one might assume, the same thing should be possible with the NHS. Conventional wisdom has it that this is not possible at the moment because the NHS is not efficient enough. Make the NHS more efficient and the managing director of the NHS will also be able to say "My organisation is OK today" on reading a few measures on a piece of paper. But this is a pipe-dream.

The fundamental difference between Sainsbury and the NHS is that the purpose of Sainsbury is well known whereas the purpose of the NHS is unclear and disputed. Sainsbury exists primarily to make a profit. The company might also pride itself on selling first class produce, not allowing unnecessary wastage, and on keeping its employees happy, but it is basically there to make money—and each secondary goal is consistent with this principal objective.

But what does the NHS exist for? Does the NHS exist to provide only medical services? Does it exist to trade? Does it exist to promote health? Does it exist to improve the population's quality of life? Does it exist to provide the raw materials for drug companies and medical researchers to carry out scientific trials? Does it exist to alleviate suffering? Does it exist to increase medical knowledge? Unlike the case of Sainsbury, where there is no dispute about the organisation's basic purpose, it is possible to find people within the NHS who would argue for each of the alternatives. And not only is it not possible to discover consensus on supreme purpose but even the most cursory survey will show that these purposes are commonly placed in a different order of priority by different people.

2. *Insufficient attention to the meaning of key words has given the false impression of consensus of purpose*

The National Health Act 1946 encouraged the illusion of a single purpose health service. The document contains apparently clear statements of purpose but, by taking the ideas of "health" and "lack of illness" as synonymous the Act fuelled confusion. The White Paper asserted that "the availability of necessary *medical services* shall not depend upon whether people can afford to pay for them . . . to bring the country's full resources to bear on reducing *ill-health* in all its citizens . . . money should not be allowed to stand in the way of providing advice, early diagnosis and speedy treatment" (my italics). Thus, in the terms of the White Paper there is a necessary causal relationship between the provision of medical services targeted against illness and the reduction of ill-health.

According to the White Paper the point of the health service was to offer medical treatment to those people who could benefit from it. Anyone with a "medical condition" could be said to be in "ill-health". Just as some people have greater medical needs than others so some people should be said to be more unhealthy than others. Nevertheless anyone with a "health need" should be able to receive "medical services" free at the point of delivery. Such a view is beguilingly straightforward, but the true picture— both in theory and in practice—is deeply confused and confusing. The confusion masked by the superficial simplicity of the 1944 White Paper (and reiterated in 1989) can be exposed in two ways.

(a) Theoretical confusion—health is a contestable term   Over the last few years discussion of the nature of health has revealed numerous alternative definitions. The definition of health preferred by the World Health Organization (WHO)[9] remains the most well known, and most notoriously idealistic. The WHO continues to take the view that health is complete physical, mental and social well-being, and not just the absence of disease and infirmity. No-one expects the NHS to adhere to such a Utopian purpose, but there is nevertheless within the service a strong belief across the professions that a decent health service should be working for something more than the eradication and prevention of disease and illness. However, the

WHO's choice is not the only candidate for the title "definition of health". Alternatives include *the capacity for a person to be economically productive, the ability of a person to carry on her normal social function, the capacity of a person to live in equilibrium with his environment, the ability of a person to cope with the mental and physical problems of life,* and still, *the absence of disease, illness and handicap.*

Clearly, whichever theory is dominant will inform the basic purpose of the NHS, even if only partially and temporarily. Equally clearly, it is vital to establish a consensus on NHS purpose if only because of the massive practical implications. Dependent upon which definition of health is most popular there may be massive differences in the process of the health service.

(b) Practical confusion—the health service is more than a medical service   The NHS does not offer only "medical services" (where medical service is defined as "clinical technique"). The NHS offers counselling, advice on lifestyle, health promotion, occupational therapy, group therapy, some general education, screening services for well people, and sometimes support in bereavement. In practice the NHS recognises that health is more than the absence of disease and illness, and gears itself to offer correspondingly broad services.

3. Lack of clarity of purpose is the primary source of all ethical controversy, and ethical controversy is endemic in the health service

If there were consensus about the purpose of the NHS then there would be far less, or even no, ethical controversy in health care. If there were a clear list, in a neat hierarchy, of the agreed priorities of the health service then a great many present ethical problems would no longer be troublesome. For example, if it were to be agreed between all interested parties that a basic purpose of the health service is to *create autonomy* in individuals then the paternalism/autonomy debate would cease to be an issue. By freely offering people as much information as possible about their medical condition and its treatment, regardless of the wishes of friends and relatives, and regardless of whether or not this might make them anxious, the health service could enable people to continue to have as much control as possible over their lives. There might be exceptional individuals for whom a policy of disclosure would lead to "psychological damage" but a health service worker inspired by the overt principle *create autonomy* would have to be convinced that deceit would ensure more individual control than telling the truth.

To take a further example, if a basic purpose of the NHS were to be agreed to be the *maintenance of a quality of life acceptable to the patient,* rather than the *prolongation of life,* then, if a person's quality of life were to fall below a level acceptable to him, the cessation of treatment would not be controversial (at least according to the overt health service remit) even if it led to the death of the person.

Such ethical issues are complicated, and no satisfactory discussion of the paternalism/autonomy and euthanasia debates can be given in the space of a page. But this is not the intention. The point is that such ethical dilemmas would be resolvable according to reference to a clear statement of purpose by the NHS. This is not to say that outside the *purposive health care system* these dilemmas would disappear, only that they would be solved within it.

There are far more ethical dilemmas for doctors and nurses than there are for solicitors, accountants, generals and shop-keepers because there is so little consensus about health care purpose. Whereas doctors might worry at length over alternative definitions of well-being, managers of a supermarket chain do not debate whether the organisation should cease to make a profit for the good of its customers. This is not a meaningful issue for a business. The Sainsbury organisation does not have to face the scrutiny of academic ethicists about its everyday functioning because everybody knows what a supermarket business is for. Certainly there are unresolved questions of business ethics—for instance, how much exploitation of the environment, of individuals, or of groups of individuals, is ethically acceptable in the pursuit of financial profit? But the basic issues of what the function of Sainsbury ought to be are not problematic because the purpose of the company is obvious.

At the moment there is a proliferation of apparently irresolvable ethical dilemmas in the health service simply because *no clear statement of purpose exists.*

Two possible purposes

It is not possible in a single paper to undertake the necessary lengthy analysis of the several plausible alternative purposes of health care. However, two simple purposes can be outlined in order to indicate the importance that an influential philosophical review of the NHS might have.

What might the health service look like if either of the two following statements of purpose were to be adopted?

Basic statement of purpose one

> The purpose of the NHS is to provide medical services (i.e. those clinical processes which are the specialist knowledge of the medical profession) efficiently and without discrimination to all people who are in need of them.

If such a purpose were to be adopted there would have to be a streamlining of the NHS. The health service would exist to deal with disease and be entirely geared toward the effective and efficient provision of medical services. The present assortment of health services would be cut down since it would be acknowledged that there has been too much diversity of function. For example, any aspect other than the clinical elements of hospice care, health education, and counselling would not have a place within a health service inspired by this basic purpose.

Basic statement of purpose two

> The purpose of the NHS is to improve the quality of life of all members of the population who might be helped.

If this purpose (which is in line with the WHO's definition of health) were to be adopted there would, first of all, have to be agreement about what is meant by quality of life. However, for the purposes of this brief discussion it can be assumed that agreement has been reached, and that quality of life is taken to involve two basic components: (a) knowledge, and (b) the capacity and actual ability to experience pleasure.

The more knowledge and pleasure had by a person the greater that person's quality of life. Category (a) is to take precedence over (b) where there is any conflict.

Applying these purposes

Angus's ankle   Unless workers in the health service are clear about the purpose of the service they will be confused about what their practical attitude ought to be. That is, they will be uncertain how they should behave towards their patients. Adoption of one or the other of the basic statements would produce different attitudes, different policies, and would have different resource implications. Take even the simplest example—a case of a person with an injured ankle attending an Accident and Emergency Department of a large hospital for treatment. Angus has been playing basketball and, in a collision with another player, has damaged his right ankle. The ankle swelled to twice its normal size almost instantaneously. Angus is in considerable pain and unable to place any weight on the injured limb. Angus fears that the ankle is broken, although the pain is not nearly so severe as the pain he experienced when he broke a bone three years ago. A friend takes Angus to the Accident and Emergency Department.

Treatment in accordance with purpose one   On attending the Accident and Emergency Department inspired by *purpose one* Angus is seen immediately by a receptionist and assigned a number. He joins an orderly queue of people sitting in blue chairs (for moderate injuries). The red and yellow chairs are for serious and minor injuries, respectively. There is no fuss, but the receptionist will not answer any questions other than those about waiting times.

The queue moves steadily into the treatment room, and it is not long before it is Angus's turn. A doctor examines Angus expertly and tells him that an X-ray will be necessary. She orders Angus to take a wheelchair. Angus would prefer to walk but the doctor insists because, as she says, walking might cause further damage: she has responsibility for his clinical condition, not his sensitivities. Angus asks, "if the bone is broken how long will it be before I can play basketball again?" The doctor replies that she is not able to make an accurate prediction without much more knowledge of Angus, his present condition and his history, and that she does not have time for this: other patients are waiting.

The X-ray is taken and it turns out that the bone is not broken, but the ankle is badly sprained. Angus asks how he should take care of his ankle, and how he might hasten recovery. The doctor says that the nurse will supply him with a support bandage and crutches, and that he is to keep the ankle elevated and not to walk on it until it will bear his weight without pain. He will have to take other advice about exercise and rehabilitation since this is not strictly a clinical matter.

Treatment according to purpose two   On attending the Accident and Emergency Department inspired by *purpose two* Angus is greeted by a receptionist who asks him how the injury happened, how he has travelled to the Department, whether or not he would like her to inform anyone else about the accident, and tells him how long he should expect to wait. She offers him a wheelchair, which he declines, and helps him across the waiting room to a comfortable chair. She explains that she will make him a cup of tea if he wants, but that it is for him to decide whether to drink it or not because the doctors might propose a general anaesthetic (in which case it would be best if he had not had anything to eat or drink for 24 hours). Angus accepts some tea and the receptionist brings over a trolley of books and magazines for him to choose from.

After a while Angus is helped into the treatment room. He is offered a wheelchair immediately, but prefers to hobble. The doctor explains patiently that this is probably not the best option. However, it is his choice. She then examines the ankle, and announces that she doubts that it is broken but advises a precautionary X-ray. When the X-ray has been taken the doctor and Angus view it together. She explains what she is looking for. Almost immediately she says, "I think you can be reassured that it is not broken" and continues to outline what she is thinking. She then discusses the management of the condition, elevation, ice, and what he is to do when he is once again able to put weight on the ankle. She asks him about his job, offers a sick note, advises against driving for at least 10 days, and suggests that this might be a good time for an enforced rest. The doctor then offers the option of seeing the resident health education officer for both routine advice and particular instruction about avoiding sports injuries, and exercising well. Angus accepts this suggestion.

The importance of reviewing purpose

These two scenarios have been described in only the most basic terms. There are obvious practical differences between them which stem from different perceptions of health service purpose. There is an indefinite number of possible purposes for the NHS, each of which would produce some change of some degree to the practical treatment of Angus. No judgment is offered about which of the two above scenarios ought to be adopted by the NHS. What is important is the clear demonstration that purpose must affect process.

Reviews of health care ought, if they are truly to improve the NHS, to shift from analysis of process to a consideration of purpose. Trying to alter process without clarification of the underlying turmoil over purpose is little more than tinkering. Only through a substantial philosophical review of purpose—a review which would have to draw on political philosophy; notions of justice, equality and equity; theories of health; concepts of autonomy; and detailed ethical analysis of all practical implications—might the health service be noticeably improved to the benefit of all. In the absence of a review of purpose there will remain:

1. Confusion amongst staff and patients about what the NHS is supposed to be aiming for (and about their respective roles).
2. Confusion amongst staff and patients over the criteria for success and failure.
3. Inconsistent decision-making both nationally and locally: it is particularly likely that decisions made by individual health authorities will not be consistent with those of other health authorities.
4. No overt overall statement of purpose of the health service, and no workable general guidelines for all staff and patients.

Given a comprehensive review of purpose the ensuing debate would eventually resolve into clear alternatives. These different visions of the NHS mission might then inform the deliberations of future reviewers of health service process. The justification for a philosophical review of the health service is similar to that put forward by the inventors of the QALY[10]—itself a measure which assumes a purpose for the health service which is not universally held.[11] The advocates of the QALY argue that at present the allocation of scarce health care resources is made according to diverse and inconsistent criteria, and that decisions are made covertly. They recognise that their alternative may be thought to be unjust by some but point out that at least it is overt, and as such is an improvement on the present situation where unjust decisions are made everyday in *hidden* ways.

A philosophical review of the health service can be justified in like fashion. There is no consensus about the purpose of the NHS. This inevitably means that decisions are taken according to a variety of rationales, some of which will be inconsistent with others. An in-depth review of purpose is required in order that all decisions made within the health service at least share a common inspiration.

Conclusion

This paper has suggested that reason in health care should be extended to include assessment of purpose as well as appraisal of function. It is not suggested that reviews of process would be any simpler given a thorough and extensive review of purpose. However, if the purpose of the health service could be clarified and agreed then discussion of process would at least be informed by a mutually understood intent. Disagreements might then take place at a fundamental level, rather than at the level of political wrangling and expedience.

Notes and references

1. I. Buchanan, MSc Dissertation. Unit for the Study of Health Care Ethics, Liverpool University, 1990.
2. K. L. White, *The Task of Medicine: Dialogue at Wickenberg* (The Henry J. Kaiser Family Foundation, 1988).
3. National Health Service Act 1946.
4. *National Health Service Reorganisation: England,* Department of Health and Social Security, NHS Management Inquiry (The Griffiths Report), DA(83)38 (London: DHSS, 1983).
5. *Working For Patients* (London: HMSO, January 1989).
6. K. Joseph, *National Health Service Reorganisation: England,* Cmnd 5055 (London: HMSO, 1972) (italics added).
7. For example: K. Clarke, Comments *passim*, 1989–90.
8. P. Strong and J. Robinson, *The NHS—Under New Management* (OUP, 1990) at p. 81.

9. World Health Organization, *Constitution* (Geneva: WHO, 1946).
10. R. M. Rosser and P. Kind, "A scale of valuation of states of illness: is there a social consensus?" (1978) *International Journal of Epidemiology* 347–357.
11. J. Harris, "QALYfying the value of life" (1987) 13 *Journal of Medical Ethics* at pp. 117–23.

Inequality among health care professionals: ethical dimensions of their relationships*

Jenifer Wilson Barnett

The common delusion that people become patients in a hospital to receive care from a consultant physician or surgeon is perpetuated by many people, not least the main beneficiaries of this view. In reality patients receive medical care without hospitalisation and it is the acute, sustained and skilled nursing and allied care which determines the need for hospitalisation. While medical interventions may be essential to change the course of illness and reduce symptoms, these cannot be successful without careful and constant monitoring of the effects of such treatment, or a great deal of psychological care and support, facilitation of physical coping, as well as the organisation and coordination of a host of services provided by others. With a collaborative and harmonious team, good two-way communication and full consultation with all participants a high standard of care and satisfaction will result.

In contrast, all too often nurses' accounts of exploitation and inconsiderate behaviour indicate that team-work is a myth and that the skills and knowledge which nurses possess go unrecognised.[1] The idea that they are victims of a system where others lead or give orders, and they obey, is quite pervasive in

---

* Throughout this chapter, for brevity, the gender attributed to the nurse is "she" and to the patient "he", with apologies to those who are rightly sensitive to this.

literature from the last two decades.[2] Enough evidence exists to assume that this picture represents reality in many settings.

Changing this situation and the behaviour which leads to it may be necessary in the future if the nursing profession is to survive and grow in its contribution to health care. Clearly a complex of factors contribute to these perceived inequalities, which need to be explored in order to rectify the balance within multi-disciplinary teams.

Nurses' own perception that they are "over-worked and under-paid" is represented in many commentaries. Clay's work[3] clearly demonstrates that this has been a popular war cry from nursing political pressure groups, even when remuneration could not be claimed to be inadequate or unfair. Collective views can only be assessed through survey of opinion or professional documents and the press but certainly Skevington's edited work[4] reinforces the impression that nurses seem to feel oppressed and poorly represented, their caring role having been under-valued and their knowledge unrecognised. Self-perception may well determine actions, and the characteristic of the nursing profession in the UK to remain self-effacing, unchallenging of others and thus continually dissatisfied and exploited leads to mass attrition and waste. Positive action and a more confident, knowledgeable profession must be created if nursing is to survive as a discipline.

However, it is not only nurses themselves but other groups within the health service who seem to reinforce the idea that nurses do not have equal rights. Chenovert's analysis[5] of professional rights (or the relative lack of nurses' rights) highlighted the fact that most employees and consumers within the hospital setting, in particular, could make demands on the nurse, who had very limited opportunities to decline or make reciprocal requests.

Both administrators and doctors have been self-designated leaders of the team, the former designing policy affecting nurses' and doctors' working arrangements and conditions of service, the latter in a more informal but equally authoritative way prescribing care which needs to be undertaken by nurses. The extent to which such working arrangements have been negotiated with nurses varies enormously. In the UK there are now fewer nurses who are executives or major budget holders than five years ago, while in the United States more senior nurses have recently been promoted within major establishments as chief executives.[6] While many UK clinicians bemoaned the fact that senior nurses used to become administrators in order to progress in their careers this is no longer seen as a desirable or powerful option in the UK when unit general managers now hold the purse strings. Care group directorates, chaired by the unit manager, may or may not adequately represent nurses.

This picture is difficult to synthesise. There will always be excellent examples of equality within health care teams, of open discussion and negotiation through power sharing. Such equality should be based on respect for someone as an individual but also as a member of a profession with responsibilities and contributions. This seems to accord with most ethical values. Those who provide care and meet their agreed obligations should surely deserve the respect and consideration of those they work with. Our changing culture no longer applauds authoritarian decision-making, actions which deny individual dignity or exploitation. Yet nurses feel they have not been afforded full consideration as colleagues and that, in essence, their treatment has been unethical.[7]

Relationships between unequal partners such as the parent–child relationship (or male–female relationship) have been used to describe the doctor–nurse relationship.[8] Lack of open self- and mutual-criticism and of partnership with clear appreciation of complementary roles and responsibilities are frequently seen. This has led to nurses feeling they have failed and to resentment that decisions are often made without their input and also without that of the patient and relatives. The context of care and pressure on resources and time is sometimes a real barrier to such discussion but there are other deep-seated reasons which negate more interchange of views.

Many members of staff may give lip service to full consultation yet in reality their behaviour does not reflect these expressed views. Doctors usually say they value the nurses' opinion and need their input. However, nurses also claim to have opinions which are not heeded and that they are not asked for information relevant to the overall care and condition of patients and relatives. A recent study by Busby,[9] although on a small scale, demonstrated that within one teaching hospital a majority of one sample of consultants reported that they appreciated the nurses' (in particular the ward sisters') views and wished that these should be expressed during the medical ward round. Nursing staff agreed that it was appropriate that they should be asked and offer their views in order to improve decision-making. When observing ward rounds, however, the researcher witnessed a traditional picture where the consultant dominated the conversation, rarely asking for the patient's or the nurse's views, infrequently asking for information from them and usually directing his conversation between the medical staff. This picture was later reflected by patients during interviews where they felt they had benefited very little from the round, despite the espoused intent that the consultants conducted rounds to review progress and treatment and to teach students. Nurses, however, did not provide information spontaneously without being asked and when they were involved it was usually at the request of the doctor who needed information. It is not surprising therefore that one of the nurses reported that she considered her main role to be "to push the notes trolley". Doctors involved in the survey definitely said they wanted nurses to be included in the round but the research showed this was primarily to pass on information and orders for treatment rather than for them to be acting as full participants.

This picture is within the context of certain changes in nursing and health care generally which are occurring. These are necessary to help the quality of service provided to the consumers of health care, to ensure that the providers are empowered to give that which they agree to be appropriate and to help consumers become more aware of their own rights. At the "grass roots" or "bedside" nurses need more skill to organise their care with a more continuous and patient-centred direction. Previously task-oriented approaches meant that nurses failed to realise what individuals and their families needed to cope with illness.[10] Of late, patient allocation or team nursing, where one nurse is assigned the care of a group of patients for a shift, is more prevalent. Each nurse can become much more aware of responses and requirements, although patients' level of dependency and thus their needs for intense care still may not be met if resources or staffing are inadequate. This type of organisation at the ward level does, however, enable the nurse to set priorities and agree goals with those she cares for.

If this continuity of care is developed further, primary nursing may be established, where one nurse will see herself accountable for the continued planning and administering of care for a small group of patients, aided by a number of associate nurses. Just as a consultant physician is seen to be accountable for the medical care of those admitted into hospital "under him" so a primary nurse is seen to be most responsible for the provision of nursing care. This logical step is now found to be successful in several units throughout this country. It is, of course, a complex change for many ward staff, not least the ward sister who was formerly "in charge" of all patients' nursing care. Manley[11] has evaluated primary nursing in an intensive care unit, finding various advantages for patients and their families, but this type of research attempting to assess outcomes for patients, relatives and nurses is extremely challenging.[12] Philosophically, a change in thinking and a professional orientation and sense of responsibility is necessary among nurses and doctors. It assumes that the primary nurse is fully informed of all those aspects relevant to "her" patients and prepared to be culpable for error or omissions in nursing care. Likewise it assumes that doctors will be prepared to accept primary nurses, with their right of autonomy, to plan care and set goals with the patient and his family and to relinquish the rather special relationship they had developed with the ward sister or charge nurse.

Not only the organisation, but the type of care believed to be effective and therapeutic, is changing. It is increasingly obvious that those who are sick often have chronic conditions for which new life skills and coping abilities are required. Nursing staff not only give care they must also help to enable an individual and his family to know about the care they will require at home and about measures which will prevent further illness or crisis.[13] They must become facilitators or counsellors, assisting others to identify and solve their health problems by gaining sufficient knowledge, motivation and energy. This is a complex and challenging role which requires great skill, education and intellectual ability.

Recognition of this enhanced responsibility and accountability within the nursing profession has perhaps led to more conflict, both personal and inter-professional. Heightened awareness of what ought to be and a lack of preparation and confidence to become health promoters may leave nurses even more dissatisfied. Reforms of nursing education[14] aim to provide an improved foundation for nursing studies, by linking schools with colleges of higher education. Nurses will not only have a better educational course but their practical experience will be clearly supervised. They will no longer provide "labour" for the wards but will gain skills through carefully planned clinical placements during their course.

In short, the solution to falling recruits and increasing numbers of leavers was to support nurses through better education. All this leads the observer to see increasing professionalisation in order to buffer the effects of subordination to others by providing a body of knowledge and of functions which justifiably can be called nursing.

Whether this will aid relationships or not remains to be seen. Anecdotally, it does seem that highly able, well-prepared graduates of nursing manage to assert themselves in the clinical setting, and other professionals adjust rather well when asked to explain decisions or consider alternatives. However, nationally it will still be necessary to support those who battle with inconsiderate treatments for patients, families and for themselves.

Recently the United Kingdom Central Council for Nurses Midwives and Health Visitors issued the fourth in a series of Advisory Documents entitled "Exercising Accountability".[15] This aims to supplement the code of Professional Conduct and provide guidelines for practice. It marks a watershed in professional standards setting, many of which concern the nature of handling difficult ethical dilemmas. At page 18 of the document a summary of the principles upon which the guidelines are based is given:

H. Summary of the principles against which to exercise accountability

1. The interests of the patients or client are paramount.
2. Professional accountability must be exercised in such a manner as to ensure that the primacy of the interests of patients or clients is respected and must not be overriden by those of the professions or their practitioners.
3. The exercise of accountability requires the practitioner to seek to achieve and maintain high standards.
4. Advocacy on behalf of patients or clients is an essential feature of the exercise of accountability by a professional practitioner.
5. The role of other persons in the delivery of health care to patients or clients must be recognised and respected, provided that the first principle above is honoured.

6. Public trust and confidence in the profession is dependent on its practitioners being seen to exercise their accountability responsibly.
7. Each registered nurse, midwife or health visitor must be able to justify any action or decision not to act taken in the course of her professional practice.

Accountability is seen as an integral part of professional practice. Upholding standards and adhering to statutory guidelines should safeguard the well-being of those subjects who receive care. In the course of giving nursing care, judgments need to be made for which a nurse is held accountable. She is accountable to the patient or client as well as to her employer, but ultimately to the UKCC, the regulatory body responsible for professional standards nationally.

Section C (at page 8) of this small, yet important, document advises that nurses must make appropriate representations about the environment of care:

(a) where patients or clients seem likely to be placed in jeopardy and/or standards of practice endangered;
(b) where the staff in such settings are at risk because of the pressure of work and/or inadequacy of resources (which again placed patients at risk); and
(c) where valuable resources are being used inappropriately.

Communications about endangered standards to those responsible for allocating resources are essential in order to rectify the situation but also to ensure that individual practitioners are not found guilty of negligence or misconduct. Silence in such situations is deemed clearly wrong. Careful records of any poor resourcing and the effects on clients should be kept and used to press for additional funds or staff.

Conflicts with managers may well result from such action but nurses now have the documented support of their regulatory body to take action based on their professional judgment on what is safe. Experience of those ward staff who have used records of inadequate staffing has shown that managers are more generous with allocation.[16] They too can use such reports as evidence when negotiating for their establishment.

The nurse is, of course, primarily responsible for providing adequate information for all decisions requiring consent. Indeed, as all aspects of care require consent it follows that patients and nurses need to hold full discussions on all relevant events. In the case of another health care professional providing inadequate explanation, the guidance is quite clear. It is beholden on the nurse to draw this to the attention of the other member of staff and seek to remedy the situation. A practitioner may also feel unable to participate in any procedure which she feels has not been fully explained to a patient or client, such that fully informed consent had not been obtained. This action should be taken only after communication with staff involved, away from the patient. The UKCC see this strategy as supportive of the other practitioners preserving them from future complaints or charges of assault.

Truth or full information should not be withheld from patients. Any member of staff who, in exceptional circumstances, makes the judgment that partial explanation is best for the patient should be able to justify this. This is recognised to be an area of potential conflict. Open discussion and a good trusting relationship should promote agreed approaches to truth telling, so the UKCC believes.

This leads on to the council's guidelines on advocacy as an integral part of the nurse's role. As part of being accountable for the total well-being of the patient it may be necessary to represent his views in the face of others which conflict. Many other professionals may also act as the patient's advocate. In this case, it will not be difficult to discuss what the patient wishes, ensuring those wishes are accurately represented if he is unable to do this himself.

Controversy over the role of nurse as advocate abounds[17] and the implication, which is perhaps offensive to others, is that the patient needs an advocate against others, such as doctors. However, nurses themselves may not be very diligent advocates if their role in team decision-making seems to be weak in some areas.[18]

In order to rectify the impression that this document is confrontational a section on collaboration and cooperation in care is included. This recognises the importance of team-work and complementary roles. At page 14 it states that a spirit of collaboration may, however, be destroyed if:

(a) individual members of the team have their own specific and
     separate objectives;
     or
(b) one member of the team seeks to adopt a dominant role to
     the exclusion of the opinions, knowledge and skill of its other
     members.

Agreement on these principles of professional practice between
the UKCC and the General Medical Council is very encouraging,
both bodies valuing the importance of open colleagueship. This
is vital to avoid harm to the patient and conflict among the staff.
It is this spirit of collaboration which staff must work so hard
to engender, particularly when some leadership styles are
inappropriate. However, it may also require substantial shifts in,
or at least sharing of, belief systems and philosophies of care.
Directions for developing better standards of practice may also
depend on the practitioners' abilities to visualise their roles
clearly and really value each other's contribution. At the heart of
such discussions rests the meaning of "professional behaviour".
For some this behaviour may not be seen as a positive advantage
to those who are recipients of "professional" care.

Professions have been viewed with scepticism by some,[19] who
feel that their members work to create elite groups who can
demand high fees and have a mastery over a vital area of
knowledge or practice. This may be epitomised by the jokes about
rich lawyers and doctors, particularly in the US. Clients frequently
complain about the charges for services, which leads to antipathy
towards such occupations and ultimately possibly a lack of
respect and to measures breaking their monopoly on particular
areas of practice. Perhaps more neutral attributes of the
professions are self-regulation by members of their profession in
order to sustain standards of intake and education, but also for
deciding on the basis for elimination from the profession (or
being struck off the register).

Specific behaviours accorded to professional groups also have
some positive and some negative characteristics. In order to
preserve a position of respect and to be entrusted with matters of
great personal significance to clients, the professional should
follow a code of conduct. Such principles as the primacy of
patient or client in health care, of keeping confidences and of
treating with respect to maintain dignity are usually represented

in such codes. However, it is those behaviours which are less attractive which lead to the mistrust and scepticism. The cohesion and collaboration achieved within many professions, such as medicine, serves their members well; however, it also leads them to appear as a rather impenetrable club where outsiders are not welcome. Inevitably this tends to indicate that such a group possesses a superiority and control over a vital resource. Any member of such a group would have to work extremely hard to convince their clients that they themselves did not perceive their own position as superior.

In the hospital setting some of the negative "professional" features tend to be perpetuated, not only by doctors but by the system which has been built up around the contribution of medicine as the most important area of expertise. The doctor's round epitomises this image that the consultant leads his teams, makes judgments and gives orders. He is the one who is being consulted, from whom all around can learn and who determines the workload of others. However democratic this consultant would wish to be, it is difficult to change interaction when so many people expect such an overt leadership style to be perpetuated. Unfortunately there are subservient, non-assertive staff who are not encouraged to be more participatory and there are also rather nervous, diffident patients and relatives who are prevented from benefiting fully from such a consultation by the unusual setting and apparently enormous authority of this chief physician.[20]

It is, therefore, important that professionalisation within the other allied professions does not fall into the trap of perceived self-importance and behaviour indicating exclusivity and superiority. Using the more positive features of professional behaviour, such as those achieved by the UKCC, there are important messages for aspiring members of the nursing profession. As equality and dignity in treatment is highly valued in our society and by nursing authors,[21] it would be paradoxical to seek to emulate the conventional models of some previous professions. Nurses must not seek to build knowledge in order to render themselves indispensable, but to give this to others and to share these aspects of their craft with those in need.

Participation in care, in decision-making and in the coordination of others' work is seen to be necessary and desirable for many patients and clients and their families.[22]

Evidence that this can be developed and that relatives, in particular, need much more help and encouragement to share in this way exists.[23] This open partnership would be destroyed by assuming that the nurse (or doctor) had all the relevant knowledge and "patient teaching" research has demonstrated that interactive small group sessions are much more effective than formal sessions for people attempting to adjust to illness or long-term health problems.[24] Nurses or other health carers may need to facilitate such discussions but it appears to be the subjects themselves who identify their own strategies, requesting information rather than being given that which appears to be most needed to the so-called professional.

It is this changing perspective on what is needed which should determine how professions and in particular health carers behave. Paternalistic attitudes to consumers and each other in the team are inappropriate to current values.[25] Respect for each other's views and knowledge combined with the overriding consideration for the primacy of the patient's well-being and wishes should determine future team-work and relationships. Although few would disagree with this, their behaviour belies these beliefs in certain situations.

Coupled with this "partnership" philosophy is the positive attitude of self-criticism and evaluation. Standards can only be maintained and improved if staff question themselves and others on whether they could do better. Currently standard setting and clinical audit is being encouraged throughout the health service.[26] This is probably most effective when the multi-disciplinary team set goals together and evaluate performances on the total provision of care.[27] Such an exercise calls for negotiation, agreement and assessment of standards across disciplines. This would involve all members of staff in peer group evaluation. Nurses would need to be strong enough to receive criticism and to discuss barriers to achieving standards when this is relevant. It also implies that individuals would need to evaluate their own care and involve patients and their friends and relations in this activity. Without this type of approach to improving standards, treatments may become inappropriate and unquestioned. One of the main justifications for the rewards of professionalism lies in accepting this process and willingly subjecting one's practice to others' scrutiny on a formal and reciprocal basis.

Central to the problem of inequality or subjugation of nurses is the non-assertive self-effacing behaviour of many British members of this profession who feel over-burdened with the increasing work-load, poor staffing levels and perceived poor support from nurse managers.[28] More awareness and discussion of conflicts and grievances may help nurses to prevent their own dissatisfaction and disregard from others. Chenovert's guidance[29] on helping women, in particular, to become more open and expressive of their feelings and opinions is pertinent to this debate. Her bill of rights includes the freedom to:

— determine one's own priorities,
— ask for resources required,
— refuse requests without feeling guilty,
— make mistakes and be responsible for them,
— give and receive information as a professional,
— help in the best interests of the patient and his family,
— question others who give care,
— be a patient advocate or help patients themselves to be self-advocates.

This list, which may include some duties and rights, reflects many of those principles contained within the UKCC's recent advisory guidelines. Essentially they help to provide the basis of independent practice but only touch on relationships within the team. They do assume that health carers have the ability to question others and defend their actions and Chenovert's book then goes on to encourage the type of interaction which facilitates this skill.

Assertiveness training has not always been seen positively and this is usually due to a misunderstanding of the principles and rationale involved. Certainly it "permits" individuals to state how they feel about a particular situation and does not discuss the subjective statement which is based on what "I feel". However, it also discusses the wisdom of compiling reasoned arguments and evidence to help a particular case or opinion. Professional communications should allow interchange of views and information which are clearly and succinctly expressed. Questioning of opinions should also be done in such a way that does not belittle the other person. Adult conversation should be non-aggressive even when strong conviction or commitment is involved. It also excludes emotional outbursts which make others feel uncomfortable, or even worse, which do not represent the point well and possibly thereby reduce the quality of decision-making. Thinking carefully through the grounds on which views should be expressed is necessary to avoid feelings of inadequacy and a deterioration in professional relationships.

Some clinical settings may already enhance assertive intelligent relationships among the team and it is these examples which encourage newcomers and consumers to be relaxed about expressing their views. However, in other settings, frequently those which are more acute, highly technical and overburdened it is difficult. Hurried "rounds" and decision-making seem to prevent team members contributing their views and problems arise which then need careful handling because they have evoked conflict or an enduring situation which is problematic for nurses and possibly others too.

Without practice and confidence it is quite difficult to change traditional behaviour and become more outspoken and questioning. Chenovert and others certainly recognise this. However, successes lead to more practice and it is difficult for others not to respond positively to truly assertive communication. Progressive "exercises" are suggested and careful planning and rehearsal is recommended. Individuals, developing these skills, gain strength but must also constantly remember that this is ultimately for the benefit of patients and clients. It is perhaps a secondary gain that this makes one feel better about the possible contributions made and recognition received as a consequence.

Partnership or team-work in care raises important questions about equality of consideration and respect. Leaders within the team may exist when one person's expertise is most needed for a particular situation. However, this must not be assumed at any time or imposed on a group where it is not acceptable or appropriate. When making medical decisions the most senior clinicians may have all the relevant information and knowledge required to do this with the consumer. For the many other multifaceted decisions that are required in health care a nurse or social worker may be in that same position. Generally it is most appropriate to consider many angles of a complex problem and different perspectives are usually helpful and should be sought.

As each member of the team develops expertise and confidence their own accountability and contribution should become clear. Patients and their families are central to these deliberations and more time than is often given is needed for a full exploration of their wishes. Through this clearer and more open method of communication the treatment received by different team members is more fair and the nature of the decisions more representative and reflective of what should constitute relevant and good care. Not only is equality among the team justified and ethically sound, it is also essential when disputes of an ethical nature require resolution.

Notes and references

1. J. E. Lynaugh and C. M. Fagin, "Nursing comes of age", in C. A. Lindeman and M. McAthie eds, *Nursing Trends and Issues* (Pennsylvania: Springhouse, 1990) pp. 27–38.
2. M. J. Johnstone, *Bio Ethics—a Nursing Perspective* (Sydney: W. B. Saunders/Baillière Tindall, 1989).
3. T. Clay, *Nurses: Power and Politics* (London: Heinemann Nursing, 1987).
4. S. Skevington, *Understanding Nurses: The Social Psychology of Nursing* (Chichester: John Wiley & Sons, 1984).
5. M. Chenovert, *Special Techniques in Assertiveness Training for Women in Health Professions* (New York: Mosby, 1987) p. 198.
6. R. B. Spitzer and M. Davivier, "Nursing in the 1990's: expanding opportunities", in C. A. Lindeman and M. McAthie eds, *Nursing Trends and Issues* (Pennsylvania: Springhouse, 1990) pp. 76–81.
7. J. Wilson-Barnett, "Limited autonomy and partnership: professional relationships in health care" (1989) 15 *Journal of Medical Ethics* 12–16.
8. L. I. Stein, "The doctor–nurse game" (1967) 16 *Archives in General Psychiatry* 699–703.
9. A. Busby, The Nurse's Role in the Medical Ward Round. BSc Research Dissertation (1990). Nursing Studies. King's College, London.
10. V. Henderson, "The concept of nursing" (1978) 3 *Journal of Advanced Nursing* 113–30.
11. K. Manley, *Primary Nursing in Intensive Care* (Harrow: Scutari, 1989).
12. J. Maguire, "An approach to evaluating the introduction of primary nursing in an acute medical unit for the elderly. ii Operationalising the principles" (1989) 26 *International Journal of Nursing Studies* (number 3) 243–60.
13. J. Wilson-Barnett, "Nursing values: exploring the cliches" (1988) 13 *Journal of Advanced Nursing* 790–6.
14. United Kingdom Central Council for Nurses, Midwives and Health Visitors, *Project 2000—a new preparation for practice* (London: UKCC, 1986).

15. United Kingdom Central Council for Nurses, Midwives and Health Visitors, *Exercising Accountability: A UKCC Advisory Document* (London, 1989).

16. B. Gilchrist, personal communication, 1989.

17. M. J. Johnstone, supra note 2.

18. A. Busby, supra note 9.

19. A. Etzioni, *The Semi-professions and their Organisations: Teachers, Nurses and Social Workers* (New York: The Free Press, 1969).

20. A. Busby, supra note 9.

21. M. J. Johnstone, "Professional ethics in nursing: a philosophical analysis" (1987) 4 *Australian Journal of Advanced Nursing* (number 3) 12–21.

22. S. Brealey, *Patient Participation: the Literature* (Harrow: Scutari, 1990).

23. I. J. Brooking, "A survey of current practices and opinions concerning patient and family participation in hospital care", in J. Wilson-Barnett and S. Robinson eds, *Directions in Nursing Research* (Harrow: Scutari, 1990).

24. K. Dracup, A. Meleis and P. Edlefson, "Family focused cardiac rehabilitation: a role supplementation program for cardiac patients and spouses" (1984) 19 *Nursing Clinics of North America* (number 1) 113–24.

25. J. Wilson-Barnett, supra note 7.

26. Department of Health, *Working for Patients, Working Paper. Contracts for Health Services: Operating Contracts.* (EL(89)MB/169) (London: HMSO, 1989).

27. A. L. Kitson, *A Framework for Quality: A Patient-centred Approach to Quality Assurance in Health Care.* RCN Standards of Care Project (Harrow: Scutari, 1989).

28. R. Waite and R. Hutt, *Attitudes, Job and Mobility of Qualified Nurses: A Report for the Royal College of Nursing.* Report No. 130 (Brighton: Institute of Manpower Studies, 1987).

29. M. Chenovert, supra note 5.

Is there a future for a National Health Service?

Trevor Clay

I want to examine an issue at the centre of public debate, an issue which goes to the heart of our perception of the shared values on which our society rests—"Is there a future for a National Health Service?"

I am going to take the perhaps unusual step of answering the question at the outset—my answer is "yes", a resounding, unequivocal "yes". The answer has to be "yes" because the alternative is monstrous in humanitarian terms, wasteful in economic terms and unthinkable in political terms.

I am acutely aware that we are debating the continuation not of *the* National Health Service, but *a* National Health Service. The question is a tacit admission that we are already locked into a process of change so fundamental and so rapid that it is irreversible. The old National Health Service, as we have known and cherished it, is going.

Before we begin to mourn its passing, however, I want to assert my belief that there *is* still scope for renewal. Where there is life there is hope, as the old saying goes, and the National Health Service remains a vital part of our national life.

The National Health Service is a uniquely popular national institution. It has been argued that "every society throws up some vast edifice that, while having some practical use, is also a pre-eminent symbol of its values and beliefs. The ancient Egyptians . . . had their pyramids. Our mediaeval ancestors had their great cathedrals. And in 20th century Britain we have the National Health Service."[1]

It is not a difficult task to analyse the reason for the health service's enduring popularity. The NHS is the concrete expression of the post-war social consensus. For a society whose shared experience of the trauma, folly and waste of war had inspired a desire for greater equity and greater equality, the National Health Service became the cornerstone on which our hopes of a better life were built.

It is more difficult therefore to understand why any government should seek to tamper with it, let alone dismantle it. The National Health Service spells powerful electorate trouble to any party or government which fails to convince the people that the NHS truly *is* safe in its hands.

Re-reading journal articles from July 1948, I am struck by the almost breathless excitement with which they were written. They read like a collective sigh of relief that better times are coming.

This example comes from the *Nursing Times* of 3 July 1948. The new NHS:

> will affect everyone: it sets out to be a comprehensive service made possible by the state for its citizens, not as a form of charity, but as their right. The cost will be borne by the state, so that none need lose their health, vitality and happiness through their inability to meet the extra expense which illness has meant in the past.[2]

There is a powerful folk memory of the bad old days which no government should disregard. It has been revived recently as vulnerable people—families with chronically sick children and elderly people—have found themselves summarily removed from their GP's practice list. The fear of being unable to pay has been translated into a fear of being denied access to health care. It heralds big problems for whomever is considered responsible. I suspect that the mud will stick fairly evenly to both Government and doctor in this instance.

I know and I acknowledge that it is not the Government's intention that anyone should be denied treatment on cost grounds. I acknowledge furthermore that the Government has explicitly asserted its commitment to the founding principles of the National Health Service. ''The NHS will continue to be available to all, regardless of income, and to be financed mainly out of general taxation.''[3]

I have never subscribed to the conspiracy theory of history. I am not (yet) so cynical as to believe that these assurances of a commitment to the principles of the NHS are mere political sleight of hand concealing a ruthless determination to dismantle and destroy. Certainly I accept the sincerity of William Waldegrave, the present Health Secretary's reasonable commitment to the National Health Service.

But those responsible for the current changes—and they include Government, free market ideologues like the Centre for Policy Studies and those general managers and consultants who have scrambled to embrace the new orthodoxy—have a very different vision of the National Health Service from my own. My vision does not accept that it should ever be legitimate to subject the sick and the vulnerable to market forces.

At the heart of the Government's proposals to encourage self-governing trusts and to promote competitive tendering for clinical services is a simplistic belief in the effectiveness of the competitive spur as an agent for higher standards. I would argue that this belief is at best misplaced, at worst, dangerously illiterate. Even if the health service could be made to function as a true market, and I do not believe that it can, the human cost would be too great.

It may be acceptable for inefficient businesses to go to the wall. It is morally reprehensible to apply the same crude mechanism to health care.

In an interview with Mary Goldring broadcast on Channel 4 in October 1989, Kenneth Clarke, then Secretary of State for Health, stoutly maintained that hospitals would pull their socks up and improve standards before reaching the point of closure. He also argued that if standards slipped too badly he, as Secretary of State, would have powers and a duty to intervene. I view that as a concession that the human price of competition could be too high. *I* say that even to countenance an avoidable slippage in standards is wrong.

I will draw an analogy with current changes in the education service. There are many disturbing parallels. Local education authorities are no longer permitted to set "artificial" limits on admissions to individual schools. Open enrolment, it is argued, will introduce market forces into education. Good schools will prosper and expand, poor ones will either improve or sink. *But you are only six years old once.* If your formative years are spent in a school which has not yet responded to the competitive spur, your educational experience has been blighted forever.

Similarly, it is no consolation to the bereaved to know that their loved one's demise features in the published league tables of hospital performance. They will want to know whether, with other priorities and better finance, death could have been prevented. We already have quite unacceptably wide variations in health performance from one region to another. Within regions there is no doubt that some hospitals and health centres give a better service than others, and are more successful. I am certainly not defending inequality in standards but I do not think that performance variations can be overcome simply through the use of competitive contracts. Loss of contracts and the consequent loss of income could simply fuel a downward spiral of declining standards and resources, threatening the viability of a unit which could have been helped to better performance.

Many of my fears about the NHS and Community Care Bill centre on my belief that a two-tier system will result from the new structures. It may be argued that a two-tier system does not, of itself, threaten the fundamental principles of the National Health Service provided that the service continues to improve overall and is free at the point of use. I disagree.

We accept that private provision is part of freedom of choice for the individual in a liberal democracy. But we must recognise that the ability of a minority to pay for private treatment does reinforce inequality in health care. I do not, however, believe that we should deliberately introduce inequality into the publicly provided health service. If we strive to eliminate the inequalities which derive from performance variations, we should not then reintroduce them by policy design.

The creation of self-governing NHS trusts is just such a policy. I am heartened that so far only 80 units have applied for self-governing status.

All the mechanisms of the NHS and Community Care Bill make opting for self-governance arguably an entirely rational response. After all, all units, whether directly managed or self-governing, will have to compete for contracts but NHS trusts will enjoy major in-built advantages. They will have freedom to borrow on the open market, freedom to determine their range of services and freedom either to set preferential rates for pay and conditions or to squeeze skill mix to fit a budget.

Dr Hugh Saxon, sometime Chairman of the Clinical Directorate at Guy's Hospital and a supporter of NHS trusts, has argued that trust status offers Guy's its best chance of controlling its own destiny. He says "Opponents overlook the fact that under the government's reforms the whole service is going to be based on a system of contracts. The choice between becoming self-governing and staying exactly as we are does exist. Within the proposed new shape of the NHS, self-government offers us the greatest flexibility."[4]

I share Dr Saxon's analysis. The odds are being stacked in favour of self-governing units. But I draw a different conclusion about the correct course of action. It disturbs me that our hospitals can be seen as autonomous units to be disposed of or redirected on the whim of an elite group of consultants or managers. As the Royal College of Nursing's President, Maude Storey, argued in the presence of the Secretary of State:

"Hold hard. Our hospitals are not your playthings. They are a national asset and a community resource."[5]

The creation of semi-autonomous "cuckoos in the nest" of health provision will reintroduce the two-tier system which existed before the creation of the NHS itself. Some may have affectionate memories of elite voluntary hospitals and of the benevolent paternalism of old-style boards of governors. We should not forget the local authority infirmaries which co-existed alongside them, providing poorer care for poorer people. Nor should we forget that there are examples of a competitive market in health care available for us to analyse. They have little to offer in terms of increased cost-effectiveness and are certainly no more care-effective than our own.

The concept of separating funding from delivery and using contracts to regulate the relationship between purchaser and provider seems to have become the new orthodoxy and is likely to remain a feature of the health service whichever government is in power.

The problem lies not so much in the contract relationship as in its competitive nature. I cannot share the naive optimism that quality criteria will become the determining factors in the allocation of contracts. All experience of competitive tendering for ancillary services suggests the opposite. If cost control is effective then quality becomes the casualty not the cornerstone of the new structure. If quality criteria are adhered to, the costs escalate. The traditional economic model of perfect competition does not apply to health care. Leah L. Curtin, editor of the American journal *Nursing Management,* explains very simply why not:

> Healthcare *consumers* (and this includes both the "buyers" and the "recipients" of care) 1. do not enter the acute care market at will; 2. do not leave this "market" at will; 3. are constrained by the depth and breadth of information provided to/for them, by the *lack of outcome measures,* by often critical time factors, and by the services available to them locally.[6]

In seeking to ape the free market, we risk making fools of ourselves. A price-competitive market in the United States has produced neither cost-effective organisation nor efficient delivery. While one in eight American dollars goes on health care, as many as one in five Americans—30 million people—are without any form of health insurance. According to the *Washington Post,* corporate America faces a 25 per cent increase in health costs each year for employee insurance—leading to the now familiar statistic that $4000 of the cost of each Chrysler car is accounted for by the health insurance of the car worker. As a result, socialised medicine, as our system is known in the US, is beginning to enjoy a respectable following. For corporate America even to consider the possibility of opting for a national system of health insurance is a dramatic testimony to the failure of the market.

Americans, traditionally, have an aversion to socialised medicine. To them it implies massive bureaucracy, restriction of individual consumer choice, sacrifice of the pursuit of excellence and forgoing technological advance. Worst of all, it implies queues, waiting lists and rationing. That formidable conservative lobby, the American Medical Association, is quick to criticise neighbouring Canada whose system more closely resembles Britain's, whose high-tech facilities are less advanced than those in the US, but whose health performance as measured by cost, longevity and the incidence of preventable disease is markedly superior.

Yet, as Eugene Le Blanc, Executive Director of Policy Development for the Ontario Ministry of Health argues: "The fact that rare Americans have access to distinguished medical services, so that millions have none, seems like rationing to me. I have never understood why Americans stand for it."[7] I am certainly not going to leap to the defence of waiting lists but I do think that if we have to have rationing, ours is a more rational and more humane method.

Of course, there are other economies closer to home which appear not to have waiting lists although they do have higher costs than Britain and an oversupply of medical personnel. Many French general hospitals have introduced the "front of house" improvements which our Government, self-styled friend of the consumer, wants our health service to make (and of course I agree that our dingy, even squalid, hospitals need not just a face lift, but a major capital-intensive programme of refurbishment). French acute hospitals appear not to have waiting lists, are well-equipped and technologically advanced. But there is no primary health care service in the sense we would understand it, no neighbourhood accommodation for the elderly or people with a mental handicap, no concept of care in the community.[8]

By allowing the acute sector to dominate you introduce another form of rationing because you limit the access to health care of people with chronic conditions. Elderly people face the dubious choice of being over-treated in hospital or under-supported at home. I have a developing fear that the Government's decision to restructure the acute sector whilst neglecting the primary health agenda, coupled with its proposals for care in the community, spell the beginning of the end of access to the National Health Service for people over the age of 65. Kenneth Clarke argued that there would be plenty of units bidding for contracts for the care of the elderly and for chronic illness because these are growth areas. But they are only growth areas if need is recognised and met. The whole ethos of the contract system will encourage a high-tech, high-volume approach to services. It will be financially attractive to corner the market in hip replacements, less so to offer quality care to the elderly severely mentally ill.

Care in the community has been described by Sir Roy Griffiths as "everybody's elderly female relative but nobody's baby".[9] I fear that it will be precisely the elderly female relatives who are shunted unceremoniously between health and social services or left to discover whether the free operation of market forces has contrived to supply a quality residential nursing home nearby. The Royal College of Nursing was almost alone in questioning whether Sir Roy Griffiths was right to recommend a lead role for local authorities in the care of the elderly. It said that his proposals were fatally flawed because they failed to grasp the scale of the nursing challenge posed by the increasing numbers of elderly people in society and the qualitatively different nature of the demands posed by people with severe dementia. The College was criticised for its stance, accused of being anti local government and unduly pessimistic. It was neither of those things but it did persist in warning of problems to come. Sadly, it has been proved right. Although the College has had some success in hammering home the demographic message, Government has refused to earmark the funds transferred to local authorities for care in the community, the use of means testing has been extended and services will be tailored not to individual need but to overall budget.

Before we give up in total despair, I want to inject a note of optimism. The 1980s will be remembered as a decade of sustained assault on collective values and on the concept of public service. Individual freedom has been elevated above social responsibility and an assumption made that the hope of personal gain will be a more effective agent of change than the desire to serve the community. This rather pessimistic view of human nature permeates the working papers which explain the Government's NHS reform plans. They have been described memorably as exchanging "the language of public service for the patter of the salesman."[10]

The assault on collective values finds its most extreme expression in the triumphalist assertion that the collapse of communism in Eastern Europe "proves" the inherent superiority of the market as a regulator of human behaviour. Extreme inequality, so the argument runs, is actually a necessary pre-condition for the flourishing of a prosperous, multi-party democracy. I think it is open to question just how widely this vision of an unequal society is accepted by the broader population, but certainly the 1980s have conditioned the middle classes to seek private, individual solutions to bridge the breakdown in common services like health, education and transport. But as an American commentator pointed out "If we know anything from history, it is that when the middle class gets upset, you begin to get substantial reforms."[11] The middle classes *are* beginning to get upset—and not just the middle classes. The old style, one nation Tories are deeply uneasy about the flipside of the enterprise culture—champagne louts with car phones accelerating away from urban squalor.

We are now starting to witness a reassertion of collective values. It begins with the dawning recognition that there are problems of infrastructure which are not susceptible to an individual or local solution. It may be the influence of the Green Movement which is promoting greater awareness of the need for social cooperation and collective provision. Similarly, it is now being argued that Britain's crumbling infrastructure is preventing the market from working.

The advent of the single European market at the end of 1992 is inducing a long overdue sense of national inadequacy about our ability to compete with our European partners. The French take national pride in investing in a system of public transport which exposes our London Underground as shabby, dirty, expensive and dangerous. Both France and Germany have well-established structures for vocational and in-service training which the new National Council for Vocational Qualifications is struggling belatedly to emulate.

In short, the need for strategic national intervention is again being seen as a necessary underpinning for the market's un-doubted role in economic regeneration. As a result it is beginning to be, if not fashionable, at least respectable to talk about shared values and common services. I am old-fashioned enough to want to espouse the cause of the National Health Service on the basis of moral idealism. It fits my personal vision of a better society. But if using the language of economic efficiency means that my argument will fall on receptive rather than deaf ears, then I am happy to argue that a prosperous mixed economy, in which market forces continue to dominate, nevertheless requires national planning and national investment in certain key areas, notably health, education, transport and social policy.

A national consensus is required on the level and quality of health provision we want, need and can afford, on the value of the pensions and the quality of life we are prepared to offer people in retirement. And I believe the public is both more generous and more knowledgeable than the Government gives it credit for. There is no doubt that the public is prepared to pay more for its health service. Opinion polls consistently confirm this. There can be no doubt either that the quickest way to improve the economic management of the NHS would be to free it from the stop–go uncertainties of the annual public expenditure round.

The Royal College of Nursing, together with the British Medical Association and the Institute of Health Services Management, came up with a formula which would assure the health service of sustained investment and growth without signing a blank cheque. The formula first requires realism. Proper account must be taken of the cost of advancing medical technology and of the extra demands of an ageing medical technology and of an ageing population. Thereafter expenditure should increase in line with economic growth—a readily comprehensible formula which could command widespread public support.

People's primary concern is with the quality of their local services. It is right that managerial responsibility should be devolved to local level provided that there is also genuine scope for local consumer input to decision-making. However, it is unrealistic for any government to expect a modern consumer society to accept indefinitely major inequalities in the level, breadth and quality of service offered. It used to be axiomatic that local issues counted most. Elections could be won or lost on the stump at local hustings. Nowadays, as Nye Bevan's biographer, Michael Foot, learned to his cost, they are won or lost on TV. At the flip of a remote control button, the superior or inferior health service down the road can be brought into people's living rooms. The public will demand that a service which is paid for from the general purse is both comprehensive and comparable throughout the land.

Despite having been members of the European Community since 1973, the United Kingdom has, until recently, not enquired too closely into the health care systems operated by our Continental partners. I think that is changing. We used to say blithely that our National Health Service is the best in the world, that British nurses are the best in the world. Given a decade of under-resourcing, which has been estimated by the House of Commons Social Services Select Committee at a cumulative

£2 billion, and given the continued flight of nurses from the NHS and from the profession, those claims are no longer made with the same bullish self-confidence.

The public is beginning to register that Britain spends a lower proportion of its gross domestic product on health than any of our European Community partners except Greece. The collapse of Eastern European communism certainly does have lessons for us, but they are rather different lessons from the complacent triumphalism of the free market ideologues. As our understanding of the boundaries of Europe expands to include Poland, Czechoslovakia, Hungary and Romania, we will find the Third World on our doorstep.

The health system in East Germany has virtually collapsed because of the flight of nurses and doctors to the West. Television pictures from Romania of emaciated babies with AIDS bear witness to the old truism: "All power tends to corrupt, absolute power corrupts absolutely." I think the British public will want to help those escaping from the yoke of oppression. I also think that comparison with Eastern Europe will bring home that we are an *affluent* society. We can *afford* a decent health system. We really *should not* need to hold jumble sales to purchase essential equipment.

It is ironic that on the eve of the creation of the NHS, nurses believed that fund-raising would no longer be necessary. It has been said that: "The voluntary hospitals that have had to exist on and ask for charity in the past, will no longer have to wonder where the money will come from to meet their increasing expenses; nor to cut down on equipment or salaries for lack of basic funds. Voluntary service and gifts will be for the extras, not for day to day essentials."[12]

I do not mind buying a raffle ticket to send clean needles to Romania, especially if my contribution is matched by Government aid, but I do question whether an advanced industrial society like Britain should have children collecting aluminium cans for special care baby units or should rely on sponsored runs to fund hospice care for the dying.

The Government's ambivalence towards the National Health Service could yet prove its undoing. A Gallup Poll published on 6 March 1989 showed widespread unease even among Conservative voters. One-third of them disapprove of the Government's proposals and do not believe the NHS is safe in Conservative hands. I do not doubt that the National Health Service will survive. The public will demand it.

I will explore later the form a new national service could take. But before I do, I want to say a few words in defence of planning. Without strategic planning, local services can simply mean pockets of excellence in a sea of mediocrity. Accidents of geography and the random application of local democracy are not acceptable substitutes for comprehensive provision. Neither are constant management reorganisations a substitute for a properly funded service.

There is probably a consensus now that we need a nationally coordinated system of vocational training in order to improve our skills base. There is recognition that to replace a qualified nurse costs the NHS around £20 000.[13] But individual health authorities do not think in national terms. They want a quick fix to plug local skills shortages. They see only the *costs* of providing child care facilities, not the benefits to the NHS as a whole.

The Government's proposals will accentuate this trend towards parochialism at the very moment when the scale of the health challenge facing us demands a coordinated national response. That response must begin by freeing the health service from the straitjacket of annual, current budgets and must assure health authorities a real and sustained growth in expenditure. I make no apology for repeating my call for a secure formula for funding the NHS—a fair share of the nation's wealth should go on health. The scale of investment needed to refurbish our hospital stock and to reskill our workforce demands a long-term national commitment allied to a national recruitment and retention strategy.

There is an interesting dislocation in the Government's response to labour market problems. Its preferred solution, local pay bargaining, is gaining ground about 10 years after the moment when it might have worked. It is possible to argue that regional pay and local bargaining are a rational response to escalating pay costs in an era of labour plenty. But I doubt whether they can work in a period of skill shortages. Regional pay in these circumstances simply shifts shortages around the country and stokes an inflationary spiral of wage demands.

I resisted the introduction of regional pay for nurses on practical and on philosophical grounds. I would not like to see the break-up of a national labour force in nursing because I fear it will have detrimental effects on patient care. Many nurses are highly mobile. Currently they move around the country in search of wider clinical experience and this improves the general skill base within nursing. Regional pay threatens to disrupt that mechanism. Allied to complete freedom for self-governing hospitals to set their own terms and conditions, it could herald a two-tier nursing service within a two-tier health structure. It is inequitable for the consumer to receive lower quality care from less expert staff simply because they live in an area of high unemployment or low wages. There is a high correlation between economic deprivation and poor health as successive studies from the Black Report onwards have shown. We need positive action to combat regional inequalities in health. That positive action should start with a commitment to tackling the *real* health agenda—with a concerted emphasis on health promotion and illness prevention.

In common with the House of Commons Social Services Select Committee, I welcome the Department of Health setting national targets for improvements in public health and devising a strategy for meeting them. Regional health authorities will be required, under the new health service structure, to develop a health profile for their resident populations. The Health Minister, Virginia Bottomley, has warned them that they will stand or fall by their success in doing so.[14] That work will be important but it does not remove the need for a national programme aimed at meeting the goals of the World Health Organization for health for all by the year 2000. I read that controversy surrounds the management style of the new WHO Director General, Hiroshi Nakajima. I find it depressing that the UK and the US seem to be following their political assault on and withdrawal from UNESCO with hostility to the World Health Organization. It may be that structural change is needed, but I fear that the sniping may conceal a more deep-seated hostility to international cooperation in health care.

International cooperation invites international comparison and demands a national response. Here the UK's record is poor. In Scotland and Northern Ireland we have virtually the worst incidence of coronary heart disease in the world. We now have a National No Smoking Day every year or so. The effort and commitment which goes into these events is not negated but is strongly diluted by our unwillingness to take on the tobacco lobby. When our Health Secretary can be bundled off to Strasbourg to vote against stronger health warnings on cigarette packets it is no wonder that we also have one of the highest incidences of lung cancer in the world.

Is it not deeply ironic that we are starting to dismantle the National Health Service before we have finished building it? It was recognised by nurses and doctors as early as 1948 that a national sickness service had been created:

> The criticism is just; the treatment of sickness, rather than the promotion of health, is the theme of most of the Act. Preventive medicine is mentioned only by implication. Nonetheless, there is that in the Act *which offers opportunities of real constructive health work to those who are bold enough and imaginative enough to take advantage of them.*[15]

Those are the words of a Medical Officer of Health, John Kershaw, writing in 1948. We must now show that we *are* bold enough and imaginative enough to take up the health challenge.

Most of my remarks have been directed at the generality of the health service but I now want to focus on two groups who, I believe, hold the key to ensuring that we *do* develop a National *Health* Service.

The first group, it will not surprise you to learn, is nurses. If we accept that the next great leap forward in public health will come not from advancing the frontiers of medical technology but from promoting better health; If we accept the desire of elderly people, people with chronic conditions or with AIDS to be sustained at home through receiving skilled, quality care then we must recognise that nurses hold the key to a new health service. Thanks to the Project 2000 reforms we will soon have a glittering array of flexible, confident nurses, secure in their professionalism and ready, from their initial training onwards, to work in either community or hospital settings.

Only a mass profession like nursing can meet the demographic challenge posed by the increasing numbers of elderly people in our society who will need skilled nursing care. Nurses are credible and acceptable to the consumer. They are effective health promoters. Midwives and health visitors have virtually eliminated the health divide for children in their first year of life. If we could offer the same quality, one-to-one service across all the population bands, the results would be dramatic.

Hospitals too can become centres for health promotion—after all there is a captive market there! But that will require a radical reappraisal of the current "treat 'em quick, send 'em home sick" philosophy. And that brings me to my second key group: consumers—the patients and clients we all work to serve. The Government has titled its reform plans "Working for Patients". It has nailed its colours to the mast of consumer choice. Health professionals must adopt the same colours and forge a new partnership with consumers in defence of the National Health Service. I do not mean merely that we want the consumer to lobby and protest to ministers, although we do. I am talking about a qualitative change in the relationship between consumers and practitioners; a change which tilts the balance of power decisively in favour of the consumer.

"Quality" is today's buzz word. It has become a sub-industry in the health care field and we are beginning to see powerful vested interests in some of the approaches and programmes which are being promoted to "manage" quality. The Resource Management Initiative (RMI) is intended to improve the quality of patient care by increasing our ability to analyse the outcomes of treatment. I warned in 1989 that in the drive to extend RMI its original thrust risked being diverted away from an analysis of patient activity and care effectiveness towards the tabulation and regulation of care.

On 28 February 1990, researchers from the School of Management at the University of Manchester Institute of Science and Technology published their analysis of the pilot phase of the Resource Management Initiative.[16] They identify two types of information system: the clinically led and the finance-department led. Not surprisingly, the finance led systems dominate the field. I believe that better information systems will, in time, show positive benefits for patient care. I object, however, to the unseemly rush to make them pay dividends.

We must return to consumers, and make them the centre of our quality criteria. In the US, a new form of quality assurance is gaining ground and attracting the interest of the major insurance groups. It is called "outcomes management" and involves the consumer in evaluating a treatment's effect on their quality of life.

Despite the fact that, increasingly, we are substituting the word "consumer" for patient or client, the UK is not yet a consumer society in the American sense. Our expectations of service—and that includes health services—are too low. We find it embarrassing to complain and when we do pluck up the courage or become frustrated enough to do so, we easily slip into aggression.

Health professionals have a major task to raise consumers' expectations about what they can legitimately expect from the National Health Service. They also have the responsibility to see that they get it—with an acceptable degree of speed, comfort, dignity and privacy. But in order to make a new partnership between practitioners and patients work, a framework is needed which will guarantee quality standards. That quality framework, I believe, must be the independent national inspectorate (recently announced) with powers to set, monitor and regulate standards right across the health and community care field, in the public, private and voluntary sectors.

Currently the Government's proposals for the health service carry many of the risks and disadvantages of the US, market based system. But they have none of the Americans' highly developed systems of accreditation and regulation. This omission calls fundamentally into doubt the sincerity of the Government's commitment to the consumer. There is merit in using the words consumer and client to denote a sense of equality and partnership. But let us not forget that when we use the word "patient" we accurately describe the position of someone who is having something done to them—who is passive and who is vulnerable. Vulnerable people, as I have already argued, should not be subjected to the discipline of the market. In a diverse, contract-driven service, it is essential that we have a nationwide regulatory structure which is tough on providers and fiercely protective of standards. The inspectorate should involve nurses, doctors and the whole health team in its work. But more importantly, it must enable consumers to participate in setting standards of care.

I opened today by declaring that our attitude to the National Health Service goes to the heart of the common values on which our society is based. Active citizens are our best hope of defending, protecting and developing a National Health Service in which we can all take pride. Empowering the health care consumer is part of the process of encouraging active citizenship. The task is urgent, the challenge formidable. If we can *all* rise to it then *a* National Health Service, *our* National Health Service, does indeed have a future.

Notes and references

1. Brian Deer, *Quality and Service,* published in conjunction with the 1989 Sunday Times Best of Health Awards.
2. M. L. Wenger, *Nursing Times* (Editorial) 3 July 1948.
3. Margaret Thatcher, Foreword, *Working for Patients* (London: HMSO, January 1989).
4. Hugh Saxon, *Financial Times,* 1 March 1990.
5. Maude Storey, Address to Congress, Royal College of Nursing, Blackpool, 1989.
6. Leah Curtin, *Nursing Management,* May 1989 (emphasis added).
7. A. Eugene Le Blanc, *Washington Post,* 18 December 1989.
8. *Health Services Journal,* June 1989.
9. Sir Roy Griffiths, *Community Care An Agenda for Action,* March 1988.
10. Robin Cook, Commenting on the Eighth Report of the Social Services Select Committee, August 1989.
11. Stephen Shortell, *Healthweek* (US) 19 January 1990.
12. M. L. Wenger, *Nursing Times,* op. cit.
13. RCN Parliamentary Briefing on the 1990 Budget, March 1990.
14. *Nursing Standard,* January 1990.
15. J. D. Kershaw, *Nursing Times,* op. cit. Note 2 (emphasis added).
16. Economic and Social Research Council, PICT Paper Accounting for Patients?: Information Technology and the Implementation of the NHS White Paper, February 1990.

Index

Index compiled by John Gibson